Remembering Ida Rolf

Edited by Rosemary Feitis and Louis Schultz

Rolf Institute
Boulder, Colorado

North Atlantic Books
Berkeley, California

Remembering Ida Rolf

Published by the Rolf Institute and North Atlantic Books

Rolf Institute	North Atlantic Books
205 Canyon Blvd.	P.O. Box 12327
Boulder, Colorado 80302	Berkeley, California 94712

Cover and book design by Andrea DuFlon
Printed in the United States of America

Remembering Ida Rolf is sponsored in part by the Society for the Study of Native Arts and Sciences, a nonprofit educational corporation whose goals are to develop an educational and crosscultural perspective linking various scientific, social, and artistic fields; to nurture a holistic view of the arts, sciences, humanities, and healing; and to publish and distribute literature on the relationship of mind, body, and nature.

Library of Congress Cataloguing-in-Publication data pending

ISBN 1-55643-238-0

1 2 3 4 5 6 7 8 9 / 00 99 98 97 96

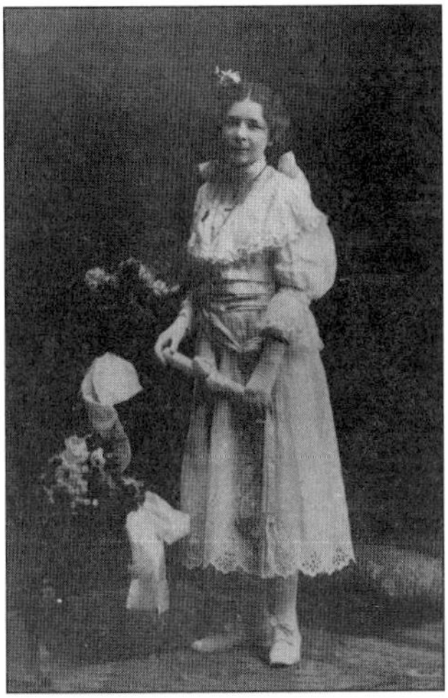
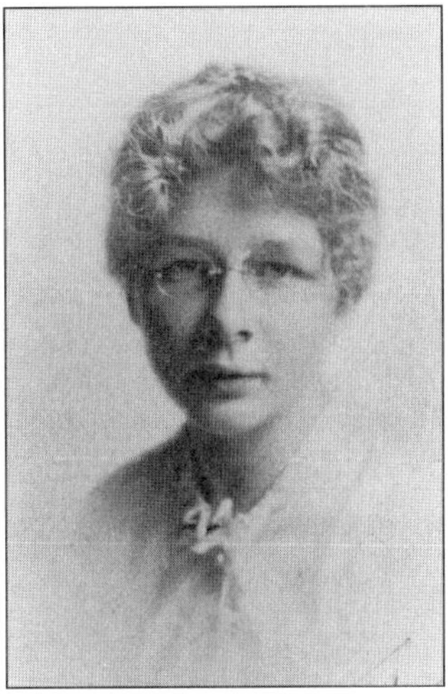
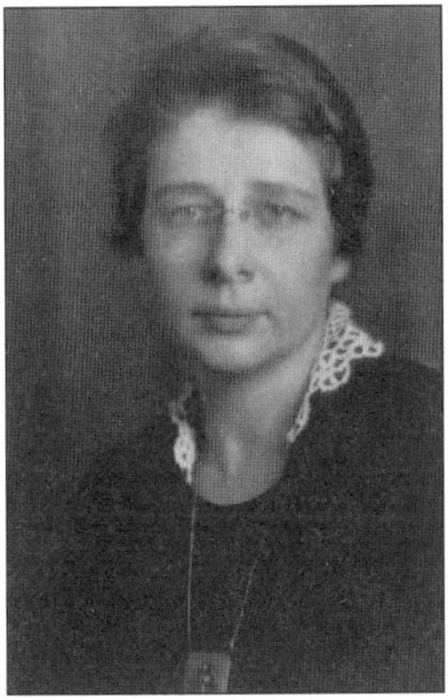
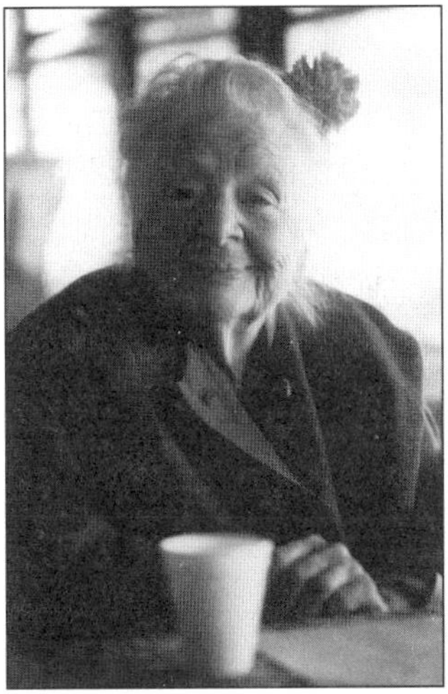

Remembering Ida Rolf

Editors' Introduction

This collection of stories about Ida P. Rolf started as a whim. We had the inspiration because we wanted to add to her centennial. We had no idea at the time that we might get contributions that we didn't like. And we didn't. . . .

The list of potential contributors came from our memories. We wanted to include those people who had been trained by IPR whether or not they were still members of the Rolf Institute. Contributors expanded our list with names and addresses we were unable to find. The Guild for Structural Integration was a major source for those people who were no longer members of the Rolf Institute. Our special thanks to Richard Stenstadvold of the long memory and excellent Rolodex. We included a few people who were not trained as Rolfers but who were close to Rolfing and to IPR.

We created the main sections somewhat arbitrarily. We assigned people to those sections arbitrarily as well, according to our memories—frequently fallible. All in all, we wrote and called about eighty people (multiple times); we received over forty responses.

Some were short, some were long. Each story tells as much about the writer as it does about IPR.

Ron Thompson rifled his extensive file for photos, for which we thank him.

Our purpose in carrying out this project has been to give people who never met Ida Rolf a feeling for who she was and what she meant to her students.

Rosemary Feitis and Louis Schultz, 1996

Early Days
(1950s to mid-1960s)

Dorothy Nolte

A Story and Excerpts from a Talk

I was visiting Dr. Rolf and working with her at the apartment for about a week or ten days. While taking a bath at the end of the day, something dawned on me that I wanted to share with her. Footwork was very uncomfortable for me. I had noticed that it was easier and not nearly so uncomfortable if I worked under water, when I was in the bathtub. I thought, I'll tell Dr. Rolf: "Did you know that the work is not nearly as uncomfortable under water?" She looked at me and said, "I know, I know." She waved her hands in the air the way she did as her kind of personal gesture and replied, "That's all I need, Dorothy, is to wear a bathing suit and work under water with a snorkel."

When I first met Ida Rolf, which was in 1957, I went for an interview in order to take her class. As you know, Ida Rolf was a one-woman selection committee

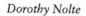

with elbows. She showed me a group of pictures. They were before hour 1 and after hour 10. She said, "I want you to look at these pictures and I want you to tell me what you see." So she went out of the room for a few minutes and left me looking at the pictures. She came back in and said, "Well?" and I said, "Well, all of these pictures go down, and all of those pictures go up." And she said, "Hmmph, you'll do." Of course, I really didn't know what I was getting into when I heard her say, "You'll do."

Ida was such a reaching person. We don't know many people who have a quest these days. When we think of someone who has a quest, we think back to King Arthur and the Knights of the Round Table, or something of that sort. How many people really have a quest? Ida Rolf had a quest and it was such a pleasure to move into that whole area of her questing. She never turned down an opportunity to hunt up a new person, to reach out and follow a new development. She was continually attempting to implement her grand design. In so doing, if a new spiritual leader was in Los Angeles, nothing would do but we'd all go down to see this new person. The whole class went.

I remember the story of the angel wings. This was

in my first class. One lady said, "Well, Dr. Rolf, you really need to hear about these people who are out in the desert—they measure your wings." Of course, Ida Rolf leaned forward in her chair, her girl's mystic was right johnny-on-the-spot and her little boy's science was back there someplace. She said, "Tell us about this," and somebody else said, "Now wait a minute, you've got to be kidding. Don't put us on, you mean we've got wings?" (I'm putting this in 1989 terms, but what came up were 1957 equivalents.) This went around for a few minutes and finally everyone settled down. It seemed that these people were flying saucer spotters who were out in the desert and measuring people's wings. Someone said, "You don't want to have anything to do with that," and Ida listened a little more. Someone said, "They're crazy," and then she leaned back in her chair and said, "Let's go see how crazy they are." I didn't go on that particular field trip, but several people did.

When Monday morning came, we all had to find out what happened with this wing thing. In that class we had a gentleman, a physicist named Bob Beck, who was and still is an electronics wizard, and of course, as you know, Ida was her own kind of wizard. Bob Beck and Ida were looking at each other and they both laughed. So we said, "Tell us, tell us, tell us." So, here are these two really world-class geniuses mentally saying, "You go first, no you go first." So, Bob says, "Mine were twenty-two feet." I've never seen Ida Rolf blush, except for this one time. And she really did, and said, "Mine were twenty-two and a half."

One time Ida said, "Well, Dorothy, which girdle are you going to do?" And I said, "Oh, God!" And a fellow student said, "No, Mrs. God." Mrs. God, I think, stuck. I really do! I think it stuck for a while; she loved it.

My husband and I took her to Pasadena to a museum—the one that holds "Pinky" and John Gainsborough's "Blue Boy." Ida had not seen Pinky before. I recall her standing in front of the painting, I feel moved in telling this, because she was truly tearful. She said, "This lifts my heart; everything in that painting goes up."

In the middle 1960s, my husband and I attended a

workshop with Fritz Perls. On the way home, we stopped at a little lake place and talked about the weekend. I saw the steps that needed to be taken to further the Rolf work in the world; this resulted in a professional workshop with Fritz during which he received the early hours of Rolfing from me. We then brought Ida to Esalen to meet Fritz and to continue his Rolfing. The rest is history. This is the source of Ida's famous statement: "Fritz came in looking like a radish on toothpicks and left looking like a radish on legs."

Dr. Rolf and I did a children's project, and out of that came the logo (of the Rolf Institute) that we use. That's Timmy! Tim Barrett is now thirty-five years old. He lives in Hawaii on the Big Island. He is about six feet tall and weighs about 170 pounds. As a child, Timmy was diagnosed with Legg-Calvé-Perthes disease. At the time, in 1959, his mother was told he would need to be casted for five years, continuously casted and recasted in order to take care of this situation. His mother chose, and this was a very, very brave choice for 1959, an alternative therapy that nobody had heard of at the time. At about nine, he started surfing. He went to Hawaii because he

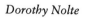

wanted to surf. He has won competition awards, in high school and on through junior college. He's married and has two children, a boy and a girl, and they surf too. He's a carpenter.

Another family member had a child about the same age as Tim. This boy had the same diagnosis. His mother chose to cast him. It's hard to say what interventions have what result. However, this boy died of a drug overdose at age eighteen, at the same time Timmy was winning championships. I thought you might like to visualize Tim with his red hair, and realize that there's a real live person who lives in the real world and he's well and happy. He has a slight limp because the head of the femur is somewhat misshapen. However, he has the balance so that he can do something that he loves with his body.

In closing I would like to say I've always thought of the Rolf work as quality control packaging. Or maybe design enhancement in container manufacturing, something of that sort. There is so much that we have to do. I think we have all done Ida proud.

Hadidjah Lamas

Exerpts from a Conversation
with Shawnee Isaac-Smith

There was an "esoteric" part of Rolfing in the 1950s. The early Rolfers used to use foot plates—metal plates on the feet—to help pull the energy releases out during the session. By the time I came on the scene, Ida had abandoned that, but if there was someone available they would hold the client's feet to help the energy release. In my early practice, we would have the client hold a small empty juice can that had been grounded with a wire to facilitate releasing.

Ida had what I thought at the time was a seemingly uncanny ability to schedule her lectures and classes at the same time there were major Subud events taking place, when Pak Subuh came to the United States. Subud was my spiritual practice and, although I did not know this at that time, Ida had once been a vigorously active member of Subud herself. I wanted to

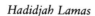

be with Ida, especially since she lived in New York and her visits to Los Angeles were infrequent and precious to me. Nevertheless, I always chose Subud over her. I did think to myself, "What an odd coincidence that these two important events keep coinciding over and over again!"

Many years later, another Rolfer told me that Ida did indeed know. She was purposely making me choose between her and Subud and remarked to that Rolfer that "Hadidjah always picks Subud." She evidently wanted me to follow her regardless and to choose her and her work over all else, including Subud. But for me it could never have been an either/or issue with regard to Subud. Keeping my spiritual connection alive was of fundamental and essential importance to me. My evolvement in this realm brought quality and meaning to my profession and into all areas of my life.

Ida did not want us to work with sick people. She wanted us to work with healthy people. She wanted Rolfing to further healthy people on their evolutionary path. In addition, it was dangerous to work with sick people—we'd get sued and the AMA would get after us and it was very scary. There was a city ordinance in Los Angeles that women masseuses had to work only on women. You could get thrown in jail for working on a man—and vice versa. It was quite a dilemma.

One time, in the 1960s, when I was rehearsing a program I was going to be performing with some other musicians, I received a surprise phone call from Ida. The thought that she had made the effort to track me down and interrupt the rehearsal made me wonder about the importance of this totally unexpected call.

It was indeed urgent. I don't remember where she was calling from, but it had to do with a racehorse that had just broken his leg. It was imperative that she have a Lakovsky belt sent to her as soon as possible so she could wrap it around the horse's leg to promote healing in the bone (and thereby save his life). Would I please do her this favor? "Of course," I said.

Georges Lakovsky was a Russian-born electrical engineer-physicist who became interested in the subject of cellular oscillation. He began by experimenting with cancerous plants, wrapping copper wire around them to create a "field," which had the effect of healing the cancer. Lakovsky's work developed out of the application of radio electricity to biology and gradually established the foundations of radio biology. Around 1923, he created the radio-cellular-oscillator; this in turn led to the multiple wave oscillator, which he used successfully to treat cancer, goiter, etc. There are many documented accounts of rejuvenation and healings.

Ida instructed me to seek out an old man who lived somewhere in the hills surrounding the desert; he would know how to make a Lakovsky belt. When I found the old man and told him of my mission, he started laughing. He pulled out some insulated copper wire, clipped it, and threaded it through a button-shaped piece of plastic. He explained that the button was necessary to keep the two ends of the wire from touching, to keep an open circuit. This was the Lakovsky belt; it could be used to wrap around the horse's leg. The old man wore several of these belts—around his neck, his wrist, his ankle. He said he never took them off, not even in the shower. Of course I started wearing one too. I sent off the horse's belt that day.

I remember in Big Sur, we (Ida and I) were having a conversation. My daughter came up to ask me a question and Ida just completely ignored her. When

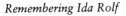
my daughter left, she said to me, "I didn't acknowl-
edge your daughter because I don't think that it's
good for children to think that they're the center of
things." She had some kind of code of how to be. I
think that this way of teaching was just her strictness.

I was fascinated by Ida's hands. They were unusual. It
was the kind of contact they had. She was really in
charge of that tissue. She really knew. People would
ask her, "What are you doing? How do you know
what to do?" She would answer, "My hands tell me
what to do." She could have answered with her
brain, talking about muscle anatomy, but she was
into feeling. When she put her hands on you, you just
knew that her hands had the ability to connect in a
way that could interact with your body and get it to
change. What fascinated me was watching her hands
working like a sculptor, almost.

Once, at Esalen, someone came in and Ida gave him a
third hour. I'm sure she did that all the time, but it
was the first time I saw her start that way. Some people would come in and she'd give them a seventh

hour to start. In teaching, she always followed the ten-hour sequence. But in practice, she'd just cut to the chase—she knew how to do it and she knew when it could be done, when the body was open enough. She once told me that the first and second hours were interchangeable, that either one could come first.

Ida once asked me what distinguished the seventh hour from all the other hours. I told her I noticed that people seemed to settle down and deepen. "Yes," she said, "that's the first time you really begin to affect the central nervous system." Then she added, "If you don't reach the nervous system, you haven't got it." This statement has stuck in my mind all these years. I believe what she meant has to do with the quality of touch. Unless you affect the nerves, you don't make a permanent change, you don't bring life to that area, and you don't change the reality of that person.

It's the higher function of the nervous system that determines what feels right to that person. At one time, she was working on me. As I lay there with her hands working under my back, I felt odd, I felt crooked. She sat back, satisfied, and said, "There, now it's straight." "But I feel crooked," I said. "No," she replied, "it was crooked, now it's straight." It took a little while, but eventually I could feel the new straightness.

Ida had an interesting assortment of friends. One of them was Colonel Arthur A. Burks, U.S. Marines, retired, and founder of the Wisdom Pool in Lakemont, Georgia. In 1958, as the result of direct experience of the "inner world," he realized he could read the Akashic records of an individual. He was also an explorer, professional writer, minister, and counselor. Colonel Burks wrote a book called *Human Structural Dynamics* about his experience of the Rolfing series, which included an exposition of Ida's theory and technique. He wanted to further Dr. Rolf's work; somewhere along the way, he also hoped he could arrange for the Marines to get Rolfed. We were horrified by the possibility, especially the women Rolfers. Just imagine Rolfing the body of a Marine, conditioned by Marine training!

Byron Gentry

I first met Dr. Rolf in a class in Dallas, Texas, in 1954. Then I followed her to Los Angeles, where she had another class. By that time, she had started to depend on me to do certain things that she or some of the members of the class couldn't do, because I had the longest and strongest thumbs in the country. So she would save the hard ones for me when I would go out to visit a new class she was holding. The next class I went to was in Abilene, Texas. She held two different classes at different times down there. I would fly from Oklahoma City to Abilene on Friday and stay Friday night, Saturday, and come back on Sunday. I did that several times. She was using me at that time as her assistant and she would have all sorts of cases for me to do that did not come regularly under the Rolfing seal of approval.

The next class was in Kansas City. She knew some osteopaths up there who got a class up for her; I went up there to that class with her. Then I went to Little Rock, Arkansas, for a class. Then I got a class up for her myself in Oklahoma City in 1958. So I had been with her quite a lot up to that time. Each time I would develop something of my own technique. I would tell Dr. Rolf about it, and she watched me grow or progress or what have you from 1954 to 1960. Eventually, Dr. Rolf went to Big Sur, California, and got connected with Esalen. I didn't see her for quite a little while—three or four years, maybe— but we stayed in contact through letters, telephone, and tapes. I would apprise her of any changes that I was doing in my technique.

Along about that time I discovered that I could diagnose or analyze a person who was not present. I could take a third party or surrogate on the table and I could check what was wrong with the person across the country somewhere by checking the surrogate on the table. When Ida heard of this, she jumped right in the middle of everything and started using me to check people that she had difficulty with. I would put somebody on the table, she would describe the condition that her client had, and I would go from there and tell her what areas were tied up. We had quite a relationship going as far as treating each other's clients.

About that time, I learned to check allergies by measuring the patient's legs. I would put the patient on the table face down and I would put a substance on their skin—on their back somewhere—that they were allergic to and one leg would contract and draw up. It would be quite noticeably shorter than the other one. Take the allergen off their back where it wasn't touching the skin, and the leg would go back to normal again. She would always have several people lined up for me. I would go to one of her classes to check their allergies and make her work easier for her because she didn't have to fight through the allergic reaction they were having to whatever it was. So we worked together quite freely that way, but she was very adamant in saying that she didn't want any psychic work in her Structural Integration teaching. She was very clear about that. The only people she had any confidence in as far as psychics were concerned were Bella and Wayne in Los Angeles and in me and what I was doing. So that's the way it was up to the 1960s.

Along about that time I discovered that I could check without having a surrogate. I could think of someone and check on their condition by projecting the thoughts about them and measuring my hands to see whether it was true or false. That was a great breakthrough because I didn't have to have a surrogate or third person there on the table. All I had to do was get my hands free so that I could get the reaction when I projected the thought. Dr. Rolf went along wholeheartedly with that. She would call me from everywhere. She was quite a traveler. She would go to China or the Philippines or somewhere in England and she would call me and ask me to check whoever her client was at that time.

The next breakthrough in my technique was being able to treat a person at a distance. I would use the surrogate to treat the person. I would have the person who was absent in my mind and work on the surrogate. The effect would be felt by the person at a distance rather than the surrogate on the table. This went on for a couple of years and then I found that I could treat people without the surrogate and be just as effective, if not more, than treating them with a surrogate.

When I found out that I could do that and Dr. Rolf found out about it, then she would call me from everywhere and ask me to check people and tell her what to do. Just on problem cases—I don't want to give the impression that she was depending on me for support because she was very self-sufficient. This was something different and she wanted to take advantage of everything she could in order to improve her technique and her ability to help people. When I got to where I could treat without the surrogate, she would call me to check a person and then ask me to treat them. Dr. Rolf, in doing this, introduced me to a lot of people and a lot of places that I had never seen and would not be likely to see. She started and built up a very, very nice clientele for me. She was very, very liberal and very, very good, and she didn't hesitate to tell people what she thought I could do.

One of Dr. Rolf's quotes that I repeat often is, "Gentry, you and I only have so much energy to give. Let's don't waste it on people who won't ever amount to anything. Let's choose the people we want to give our energy to." That is very good and sage advice because it is very true. Everyone is not ready for everything we have, so give it to the ones who are ready. Later on, when Dr. Rolf started having classes in Boulder, she had me come and speak to the classes. Also she had me come and speak to the Rolf Institute's annual meetings.

Dr. Rolf was very fond of the mountains. She liked to go up in the mountains, especially the Rockies. It seemed the nearer she got to nature, the more grounded she felt. After having had a class in Boulder, she would go up in the mountains and stay two or three weeks and get back her energy and get herself grounded. She would go up there by herself, usually in a Volkswagen. The class was concerned about her doing this. They would ask, "Dr. Rolf, what if you get up there in the mountains and have an accident or get sick, what would you do?" She said, "I'd call

Gentry," and they couldn't understand that. She was going to go to China after one of her classes and they said, "Dr. Rolf, if you get sick in China, what are you going to do over there?" She said, "I'll call Gentry." It was so unusual for anyone to say that, that some of the members of the class who lived in Florida and were on their way back from Boulder came through to see this strange character in Oklahoma City whom Dr. Rolf would call if she got into trouble anywhere. They were examining me to see if I had two heads, no head, or whatever. Several came through on a curiosity binge, I'm sure, but then we would have a session and I would explain to them what I was doing and how I was doing it.

Even though Dr. Rolf was very much interested in the psychic work that I was doing, she did not want it to be done in her classes. Yet one day as we were in the car and headed up the mountain—Mary [Gentry], Dr. Rolf, and I—Dr. Rolf, out of the clear blue, says, "Gentry, what do you think you could teach Rolfers?" Well, I drove along a little bit further, in the depth of meditation, and I said, "Intent." We drove along a little further, without her saying anything, and pretty soon she said, "Gentry, I think you're right."

From that time on "intent" was stressed in her classes. Because up until then you were just supposed to go in there and get it. Just get in there and go on down a little deeper—go in there where it is. When the idea of intent was brought up she changed her teaching to the point that if you have the intent of relaxing the structure that is down underneath there, that you're trying to get, mentally you will relax it; that's the thing that I've been saying, go down in there and get it. I didn't term it that, but that's what it is. It's your intent, your intent will do that. You need that intent before you start your manual manipulation because your intent is a very strong thing and can aid a great deal in structural integration manipulation. Dr. Rolf was not very lavish with giving compliments. She did compliment me on that, and she used it.

She used to come through Oklahoma City and stop at our place and stay two or three days, maybe a week. Mary would cook things she would like and we would sit her out in the sun on the patio in the back. I would work on her. She and Mary were very close and they liked to talk astrology and things like that. Dr. Rolf was very lavish with any new technique she came up with. She flew through here and stopped in Oklahoma City just to tell me and show me the new technique she had worked out for the psoas, and how important it was to the structure of the entire body. As I say, she was very free in giving her knowledge to me regarding these things. So we got along real, real well.

When she wasn't around we kept in contact through tapes, telephone, letters. I made a "healing" tape for her and relaxed the muscles of her back and she commented that she could feel the relaxation going on. I use the word "normalize" quite a lot. I was trying to normalize the structure and get it as normal as possible and she says, "Gentry, I don't like that word 'normalize.'" And I said, "OK, give me one that's better." She thought about that for three or four or five years and she said, "I still don't like it, but I don't have one that's better." That's the way we left it. I still use "normalize" in certain areas when we're talking about Polarity or something like that.

My psychic relationship with Dr. Rolf was very, very good. She would ask me many things that she would not ask in open class and she trusted me enough to know that I wouldn't bring it up in open class if she didn't want me to.

Ed Maupin

In the summer of 1967 I was a resident at Esalen. I heard that a certain woman had come to do body-work with Fritz Perls, that she would work with other people as well, and that those who had gone to her spoke well of her. I don't know why I was attracted, especially when she insisted on a ten-session commitment at the (for me) enormous price of $150, but I agreed and lay down to undergo the first session.

Though the work was painful, Ida clearly knew what she was doing. She kept up a continual patter of conversation, which was reassuring. Periodically she would have me stand in front of a mirror to notice how my body had changed. This was not reassuring, since she seemed to be pressuring me to see shifts I had not the visual acuity to perceive. However, her manner implied that "mamma knows best" and who was I to argue—especially with so forceful a mamma?

I have several impressions from those early

weeks. First, I was impressed with her legs. Though she was about seventy-five at the time, her legs were straight, calves large and strong and seemingly free of varicosities or other blemishes. Second, when she sat next to my reclining form on the bed I felt an aura of strength and calm. This is always my association when someone says that a Rolfer primarily transmits his/her own sense of the line. Third, somewhere in the agony of my fourth hour I realized that I was back in the state of my original "beginner's enlightenment," which I had experienced in Zen meditation and which had been my inspiration for being at Esalen in the first place. It was at the end of that fourth hour that I asked her to train me in the method. I had learned from the Zen experience that my relationship to my body-as-creature was crucial, and I was looking for a body-oriented method of psychotherapy. Her work was putting me into that state of clear witness out of the very need to deal with the intensity of sensation.

When I arrived as an auditor in her first class in San Francisco (winter, 1968), I was struck by her seeming paranoia; she kept the blinds drawn in the motel room where class was being held for fear of being arrested for "practicing medicine without a license." I was touched and amused. After all, Edgar Cayce had spent time in jail for diagnosing at a distance, and I realized how many years Ida had courageously developed her work under the shadow of that kind of threat.

That seeming disparity between the tough and the tender, between the sublime and the pushy, between genuine authority and vulnerability, continued to touch me through all the period of my involvement with her. Sometimes her speech seemed relentless and rhetorical. She always had some point to drive home. But when she smiled the light in her eyes seemed spiritual and gorgeous. Our joke was that inside her little-old-lady-suit was a Mack truck, but inside the Mack truck was a bodhisattva, an angel, a realized being. I personally experienced something of the angel once, when she pursued a particularly painful misalignment in my knee, and when I gave way to her, I felt an absolutely Conscious Presence waiting for me in her touch.

Later, when my own practitioning class took place in Big Sur, she would alternate between the radiant smile and commanding us to "get your head up" or "get your waistline back." We all sat around in painfully stiff alignment, our heads so "up" it was hard to observe her demonstrations. I was, at the time, rather a favorite, and when I remained behind after class she would confide her concerns in a touching way, in the tone of a woman needing the support of a strong man. When she came to my cabin for dinner, she refused wine, saying, "Wine is not a friend of mine." When my daughter was born Ida glowed with compassionate approval—a kind of Olympian benignity toward life, I thought—and promptly repaired something in the infant's shoulder girdle which seemed disorganized.

Somewhere about this time my love for her took a more ambivalent turn. Ida was concerned that none of her students were really getting a grasp of her work (which was true of me, I'll admit, though I could generally transmit my memory of Ida's touch). Once she called me into a subsequent class and commanded me to show what I knew of the psoas work of session five. It was a harrowing, humiliating moment, though I survived. And suddenly there were all these new Rolfers, whereas I had earlier been the favorite.

When the Rolf Institute was proposed, I refused to join. I don't remember my reasons, and later I was to regret not joining, but I feared that if I joined and later resigned, I could no longer call myself a Rolfer. Ida was angry about my resistance, and for some years I would hear about critical things she said about me in classes. It was painful for me. When I worked I carried on an interior dialogue with Ida, proving again and again that I was a good Rolfer.

This whole ambivalent period between us had an amusing resolution. At her birthday party in 1978 I saw her again for the first time in eight years. When she greeted me in the reception line I could see the shades of judgment come down over her eyes. Then Gabrielle Roth, the mistress of ceremonies, picked up the microphone and said, "Ida, words cannot express what I owe to Rolfing." She proceeded to tell us about coming to Esalen with a knee injury that physicians had told her would permanently prohibit her dancing. "And Ed Maupin did something excruciating to my knee but then it was okay, and I've been dancing ever since." I felt blessed . . . exhilarated . . . I was amazed that The Process had brought a testimonial to my work into Ida's very birthday celebration. Later, when I went through the reception line again, Ida looked at me brightly and said, "Well, are you still Rolfing?" After that, my interior dialogue with her ceased.

Robert K. Hall, M.D.

I remember Ida as a teacher of fierce commitment to her work and to her task of grounding that work in American society. She did her job. I also remember her as a lady of great compassion who carried a sharp sword. Often, I honor her memory in my heart and give thanks for the ways that she enriched my life.

I experienced my training from her in a closed room on the second floor of the Laurel Lodge Inn at the corner of Presidio and California, in San Francisco, in 1968. The drapes were always drawn and we—Jack Downing, Bernie Gunther, and myself—were told not to make loud noises. She was concerned about the possibility of someone calling the police. Her concern wasn't unwarranted, since, in those days, what we were learning was even more strange to ordinary America than it is now.

She was a powerful woman. Her relentless touch helped my five-year-old son grow out of severe lordosis. When she worked with him, he never complained of the discomfort he was obviously feeling from her radical rearranging of the fascia of his little body. He told me he could tell that she was helping him.

Later, she worked with my best friend, who had volunteered to be a model. The day after her session on his face, head, and neck, he came down with severe Bell's palsy (the remnants of which remain on his face today). I was very disturbed, and felt guilty for having contributed to my friend's suffering by bringing him into the training. Ida refused to acknowledge that her work the day before had anything to do with the problem. I couldn't believe that was so. And thus began many years of deep ambivalence about our teacher-student relationship. I wanted her to acknowledge some doubt. She refused. I became estranged from her over the next few years.

I returned from India in 1970. I had been learning meditation from a great spiritual teacher and Polarity therapy from his physician, Randolph Stone. My work with the body had undergone great change and was developing into what later became a large part of the curriculum of Lomi School. Ida called me and told me I needed to take an advanced training in Rolfing. I told her I didn't want to because I was pursuing my work with Dr. Stone at that time. I'm sure my continuing ambivalence about her as my teacher was the real reason I refused.

When next I heard from her, it was through her

lawyer. The Lomi School training was underway on Kauai. He told me that I was claiming to be doing Rolfing and that Ida demanded that I "cease and desist." Actually, I was not claiming any such thing, being much more interested in the integration of Polarity therapy with hatha yoga, movement, Gestalt, and meditation. I responded in writing that I did not consider myself a Rolfer, but that I couldn't be responsible for what others were saying.

Several years later, the same lawyer contacted me in Mill Valley and told me that Ida wanted to meet with me in her apartment in Cathedral Hill Tower. We made a date for my visit on the following Sunday afternoon. I am, to this day, amazed at the depth of my emotional transference on Ida, because I realized, with disbelief, on the following Monday, that I had completely "forgotten" the appointment and had unconsciously stood Ida up. I was embarrassed and humiliated. When I called her to apologize profusely, she said that perhaps I didn't want to see her at all. I asked her to please see me. She agreed, and we met the next Sunday in her apartment.

When I arrived, she greeted me warmly enough. We had not seen each other in many years. Our conversation was a bit stilted and tense (at least on my part). Finally, she asked me if I would like some of her favorite Israeli wine. Although I didn't drink alcohol, I accepted gladly. She broke out the wine, and we proceeded to drink quite a bit. In fact, I got a little drunk. I think she did too, but I've never been sure.

Near the end of our meeting, she asked, "What do you teach in that school of yours?" I answered with the first thing that came to mind: "Attention." She looked at me a long time without expression and finally said, "Good."

As I was getting ready to leave, she started looking at my body in that discerning and critical way she had and said, "You need some work on your second lumbar. You martial artists often need that." I politely asked if she could recommend a practitioner for me, and she gave me, without hesitation, the name of a Rolfer who had started out as a student of mine before he went off to her training. A voice in my head immediately said, "No way."

As she stood at the door to say goodbye (the last time I would ever see her), she extended her hand to me in farewell. I took it, bent my head, and kissed that hand. I have been free of struggle in my relationship with Ida ever since that moment. I add my gratitude and respect to that of thousands of others for her great gifts to me, and for the pathway she opened for many who realized the necessity for greater ease and awareness of our physical manifestation here.

The Early Guild
(late 1960s)

Mary Bond
Off to a Flying Start

It was May 1969. Emmett [Hutchins] knew I was in some kind of pain because I lay moaning in the back seat the whole way up Highway 1 to Big Sur, then the Rolfing Mecca. We were due to begin practitioner training first thing in the morning. Apprehensively we rang the bell and, though it was well past bedtime, Dr. Rolf let me in and listened to my story. I'll let my readers surmise precisely how I'd managed to get my pubococcygeus muscle into such a spasm. Ida tapped her forehead and rolled her eyes in that characteristic gesture of amazement at human foibles. Then, after rummaging around in her bedroom, she handed me a hot water bottle.

Peter Melchior
Advanced Class

It was early summer, 1972. During the first "official" advanced class, at Joe Adams' house in Big Sur, Dr. Rolf announced during the morning lecture that she had something special to say to us.

"You all saw the little tree at the side of the front door," she began. "Well, that tree is known as the 'Ego Tree.' I would like you all to hang your egos on that tree as you come through that door into class each day. You may pick them up again on the way home."

Considering the sheer weight of the massed egos in that class, it should come as no surprise that we all laughed and said to ourselves, "Good joke, Ida." I, for one, forgot the whole thing immediately. However, as the week progressed, it became apparent that she really meant it, and was going to stick by it. (I was caught twice in the first few days pursuing social interactions in class, to the raucous delight of my colleagues.)

She really was saying to us that this was an advanced class, and that one of the characteristics of the class was that we would be expected to devote every moment of class time to learning the art of Structural Integration—every moment of every day! I tried to imagine what it would be like to be able to actually remember myself consistently enough to do it, to spend not one moment in class concerned with anything unessential, to remain single-minded throughout the day for six weeks running—to give the work my full attention.

I had never even entertained such a thought before. I nearly went crazy in the course of those six weeks, trying to make it happen. This became one of the most intense periods of my life. Four days a week, I was involved in teaching a basic class; the other three, I attended the advanced class.

Dr. Rolf had said she would see me in the advanced class, and I told her that Emmett Hutchins and I were teaching a basic class. She replied, "That's only four days out of the week—you can attend the advanced class on the other three!" I already felt I was spending all my time learning the work. How could this not be enough? Was the woman crazy? Was she simply not aware of the private requirements of men everywhere?

Early one morning, as I was walking up the highway, enjoying the sound of the sea and thinking that I was for a moment free of these immoderate demands, a voice suddenly came arrowing through the fog—a voice I had come to know too well: "Get the top of your head up!"

Ida had been looking out the window and saw me passing by. I nearly had a nervous breakdown, but not until I had found the top of my head. Today I am missing that voice very much.

I have come to believe, finally, that Dr. Ida Rolf was "crazy like a fox." This one simple instruction, which suggests that it is indeed possible to remain conscious of one's intention for a particular amount of time, has stayed with me for nearly twenty-five years, haunting me. I still make the attempt, every once in a while, to set aside a period of time and to remain consistently focused on one thing, giving it my full attention; and each time, though I may fail technically, something of great value is gained— something that continues to enrich my life and make my work more effective.

Of course, none of us succeeded in fulfilling this instruction during the class—we never even came close. But I believe a seed was planted on that day and that the tree that grew from it is still bearing fruit, and I am grateful.

Another Story

Dr. Rolf was teaching a class at the Adams House, on the Big Sur coast, near Esalen. I was teaching a class nearby, at the South Coast Motel. Ida decided that I should bring my class down to the Adams House, to meet with her class during the mornings. She was dishing up some pretty heady stuff just then, and I would take my class back to the other class-room in the afternoons and try to scrape them off the ceiling and teach the basic work to them.

For this class, having long sensed that Ida had considerable disdain for my rather loose style in running a class, I had decided that I would teach the most orderly and structured class the world had ever seen (at least the world within a twenty-mile radius of Esalen). We were just marching along in tight formation and happy as clams. I knew Dr. Rolf would be truly surprised and pleased when she saw how I had turned over a new leaf.

One morning, we all showed up at Ida's class-room, and she began the morning lecture. It was on the topic of "Creative Chaos." She wove a glorious story about the requirements of creativity and the need for creative space—for letting go. As she closed the lecture, she said, "And that is just why this neat little package that Peter is trying to put together down there at the South Coast Motel won't work!"

That afternoon, I went back to the classroom and blew up the whole structure we had been using. We never mentioned this matter again.

Judith Aston

It is May 19, 1996. Today would have been Dr. Ida Rolf's 100th birthday. It was only four days ago that I told Louis Schultz and Rosemary Feitis how sorry I was not to have the time to do justice to writing something for the collection of Ida Rolf stories. I told Louis I wouldn't have time to think until August; after we laughed, Louis said, "Fine, but we'll keep calling and harassing you until you do!" So it seems fitting that I sit down to focus on my Ida stories on her birthday.

Dr. Ida Rolf was an impressive woman not only in her pioneering work in the field of human evolution and her understanding of biochemistry, but also in her willingness to meet enormous challenges in her family, in her work, and with nature. I laugh now when I remember the thirteen-day Colorado River raft trip that Greg Hayes, M.D., organized for sixteen of us Rolfers. Naively thinking this would be quite an unusual adventure for Dr. Rolf, I invited her to join us. She said, "Oh, I've already been down the Grand

Canyon" . . . pause . . . "before it was dammed."
(Enough said.) I heard Dr. Byron Gentry tell another
story in which Ida got out of the car, walked past the
flood barriers for a rising river, and led Byron to follow in his car. After all, she needed to be back in the
city for an appointment.

I had many occasions, over nine years, to spend
time with Dr. Rolf . . . shopping, eating, driving (as
well as many hours of meetings as a member of the
Board of Directors and the Education Committee).
She had quite a sweet tooth. One time, I visited Dr.
Rolf for three days after she had moved from New
York to New Jersey. We stopped at a market for a few
things, including a half-gallon of Breyers Butter
Pecan ice cream. We discovered that we each had a
specific taste preference that would quickly finish off
that carton. I liked and was digging for the pecans
with a bit of ice cream, while she would uncover the
pecans for me and go for the ice cream. We couldn't
wait to get to her house. We ate it in the parking lot.
We had such fun, like two little kids; I don't even
think we got sick.

In the spring of 1968, Dr. Rolf introduced me to
the body's *magic*. Shockingly, she could work on the
body's tissues and the body could change . . . poof
. . . just like that! What an opportunity this was. This
experience shattered my previous idea that by age

twenty-one you were the best you were ever going to get and the rest of your life just went downhill from there. Thank goodness, as I am still over twenty and still improving.

For the summer of 1968, I had the opportunity to be Dr. Rolf's Girl Friday. Maybe now I could be better at serving. Then, in my twenties, it was difficult to get all the details done correctly. There was one detail, however, that I learned from Dr. Rolf and will never forget. In fact, I have shared it with at least a thousand people by now. During breaks, Dr. Rolf would ask me to get her coffee with cream. After the first day, she asked, "Did you put the cream in the cup first?" I had not. She relayed the importance of pouring the cream first. Although I had always preferred tea until then, I decided to try her style of coffee. It was amazing. If you put the cream in the cup first, the coffee is always being mixed into the base of cream. If the coffee goes into the cup first, the cream is always mixed into the base of coffee. The second result seems more bitter or acid. Not only did I learn a basic principle of chemistry, I now drink coffee, and I pour the cream into the cup first.

In 1971, Dr. Rolf started to invite me to work on her hands whenever I was around. She had arthritis; my work gave her some relief. Over the years, her requests eventually included working on her whole body. She was appreciative and I felt privileged. It reminds me that it is a privilege when our clients give us the trust to work with them and their personal history.

I am very grateful for my time with Dr. Rolf; the good times touch my heart and continue to make me smile. The challenges of working with her made me stronger and wiser. In 1971, the Reverend Joan Mallan told me that gratitude is the mother of consciousness. I look forward to even more gratitude and more consciousness.

Rosemary Feitis

I worked for IPR for about four years, on and off. It wasn't a job, it was a way of life. Most of my memories are like that—about the odd little concerns and how we solved them. There was the flower for her hair; someone once told her she should wear a flower in her hair and she had been doing it ever since. A daily fresh flower can sometimes be a conundrum.

She liked her afternoon tea in a thin china cup, with real cream. I still feel my hand reaching out to pretty teacups that might please Ida, and she has been gone a while now. She liked chocolate-covered marshmallows, which I detest; they still catch my eye.

She wasn't a snob about how she liked to live. Simple restaurants pleased her more than fancy ones. One evening we were taken to someplace pretty special in Florida. Our host had let the musicians know that he was bringing an important guest, so they gathered around and did themselves proud. Ida listened for a bit, then asked them to stop making that noise, she couldn't hear the conversation.

Fritz Perls sent me to Ida for Rolfing; he thought it would do me good. Ida had left instructions at the Esalen desk: go soak in one of the Esalen baths, and she would call for you when she was ready. So I went and soaked, my favorite thing to do at Esalen. She called. I gathered up my jeans and tee shirt (no underwear) and went on in. No idea in my head that she might not like the view. She lit into me about the lack of underwear, and there is in existence, somewhere in the Rolf Institute basement maybe, a picture of me in panties and bra that Ida kept for just such purposes—much too large—looking bewildered but taller after my first Rolfing session.

It's a wonder I got the job working for her. Fritz recommended me, but I'm pretty sure what did the trick was a kelly-green suit I wore—with stockings and formal shoes—to some sort of Esalen celebration. That and the fact that we both had been to Barnard College. Toward the end of that first spring, we went to Los Angeles so she could give a lecture. I felt very much the dogsbody—I drove down, I lugged in the slide projector, I made sure the bed and the camera and the sheet and all of it was at hand. I made sure the volunteer had underwear. So I was somewhere at the back of quite a large crowd when I heard her calling. "Have you seen Rosemary—my secre- . . . my assist- . . . my *friend*, Rosemary?" She wanted her hanky.

Mac MacDonald was a rehabilitation physician at the Kaiser Permanente rehabilitation clinic in northern California. He was impressed with what Rolfing could do, and trained as a Rolfer. Shortly thereafter, he invited Ida to give a lecture/demonstration. The head of the clinic was an important author in rehabilitation medicine, and Ida was pleased at the chance to show discerning professionals what Rolfing could do. The head of the clinic was vocal in her appreciation of Ida's work, and altogether it was a satisfactory event. As we were walking down a long corridor toward lunch afterwards, Ida and Mac were up ahead, I was in the middle (lugging something), and clinic staff brought up the rear. The head of the clinic was explaining to her staff that the changes were truly remarkable, but, of course, they were not the result of Dr. Rolf's technique. Rather, this was an interesting case of a truly mesmeric personality who could hypnotize patients into better alignment.

Somehow there got to be the tradition that people would bring babies to Ida on her birthday, for her to work on. Probably it was because her birthday always fell in the middle of a class and none of us thought she should be teaching then. One of her birthdays came in the middle of a class she co-taught with Brugh Joy at Apple Valley Ranch. His main room there had a wonderful fireplace and very thick carpeting. It was a rainy day, and the babies ran around without diapers and enjoyed the warmth and the company. I especially remember one little blonde thing, about eighteen months old, playing with all of us, very outgoing and delighted with her new legs from grandma. It got to be time to go home, which meant diapers and clothes. All of a sudden there was a shy and clingy and sad little thing, unsteady on her feet and in her being. It brought home to me what Ida used to say about those thick wads of diapers unbalancing the child.

Ida's capacity to see into the body was legendary. We were always trying to catch up to her perception, always a little convinced there was more than visual acuity and experience involved. She'd tell us to sharpen our eyesight, there was nothing extra-sensory involved. One of my last memories of Ida is sitting next to her in a class at the time when her eyesight was getting seriously bad. "Rosemary," she asked me, "who's that over there at the table on the other side of the room?" It was Joseph Heller, one of her favorite people; and I told her. "Joseph," she said, "it's under your third finger."

Ida could be naive, especially where "higher con-sciousness" was concerned. I think she was some-times a little startled by all the adulation she got. On the one hand, she had all these people around who were awed by her abilities and her aura. But on the other hand, there was always a shortage of money and the power to do what she wanted. Her reach was always exceeding her grasp, and it made her vulnera-ble to the people who claim to draw on the wisdom of the ancients.

One such was a man named Krone (not his real name), purportedly of the Dutch nobility and lately from the Dianetics group, where he said he'd risen in the organization and become a "clear." (Dianetics is the outfit that hit the media in the early 1980s for putting a rattlesnake in the mailbox of an apostate member.) Krone was tall and blond and a smooth talker.

I was the business part of Ida's outfit at the time, so Ida turned him over to me to get him books and a roof over his head and generally prepared to be trained in the next Rolfing class. Never mind that he was ignorant of any anatomy, penniless, and very de-manding of service—he was a nobleman and a "clear" and she was going to train him.

By the time we got from Los Angeles to Big Sur, I was seething with annoyance and so were a number

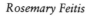

of others who had met him. How to get this cuckoo out of the nest? It took Jan Sultan's muscle and forthrightness to achieve the miracle—he packed the man's bags and put them on the porch. Then he locked the door. Ida must have been having a few doubts of her own, for she never mentioned Krone again.

Ida's funeral was in New Jersey. Richard Stenstadvold flew in from Boulder and we drove down together. We walked up the aisle together, and I was glad of his arm, because the person lying there didn't look anything like the Ida I had known. But then I looked at her hands, and there she was. Her consciousness and her life were still in her hands, just as I remembered them, recognizably Ida even in death.

Fritz Smith

I studied with Ida in 1971 in Big Sur. Of course, many things were bound to happen in such an experience, but one thing stands out particularly to me—a realization that has served me in many ways and helped to open new doors. Specifically, I had the good fortune to be Ida's model for the last seven of the ten sessions. For some reason, the gentleman that she had originally selected to be her class model needed to withdraw from the program after the third hour. It was my good fortune to take his place.

The realization, or maybe I should say experience, was that *Ida didn't hurt me while she was Rolfing me*. This was totally incongruous with what we students were doing with each other. Those other Rolfings really hurt. I was in pain when others worked on me and I hurt people when I was Rolfing them. It became expected that a session would be painful because that was what Rolfing was. It was par for the course.

It was only later, especially after I began to study

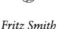

acupuncture and learn about energy, that I developed a perspective on what happened in those sessions with Ida. I believe that she was actually working with energy during the Rolfing session, but did not have the vocabulary at that time to recognize that possibility or to teach it. Acupuncture and energy generally had not yet become household words, and the energy concepts were not yet in the collective mind field.

Specifically, I believe that Ida would develop or create a bolus of energy in front of her finger or elbow. As she would make a pass through the fascia, this bolus would precede her physical body, opening the energy field ahead of her physical arrival. I would feel the pressure of her physical structure, but not pain.

Had the concept of energy been in common vocabulary in the early 1970s, I think that Ida might have taught Rolfing somewhat differently. Rolfing might not have been known for its pain. I think she was doing something beyond what she was teaching, and didn't have the words to explain it.

She showed me a world of possibility, of envisioning energy as different and separate from structure. I learned from her that they influence each other in every moment of our lives. Thank you, Ida Rolf.

Hector Prestera

In my first class with Ida, in Los Angeles, which I audited, she kept me sitting and watching, always challenging my M.D. mind with its fixed notions of anatomy. I really wasn't seeing body parts moving as Ida suggested. I looked and looked, remaining both skeptical and frustrated. Finally one day as Ida said, "Now look at how the space between the ischial tuberosities is going to widen," I looked. And then it happened! I saw the space between the tuberosities widen—I was astonished. It really happened. Ida changed my way of looking at the world forever.

In a class in San Diego (I was now several years into Rolfing), Ida asked me to help teach. I was honored by this and feeling a bit of "Well, I have gotten the hang of this." I and another Rolfer, a rather powerfully built colleague who was practicing in Santa Barbara at that time, were trying in vain to create some movement at the sacrum of a client who was himself very muscular, with generally dense and thick connective tissue. So we worked and worked on this poor man's pelvis, desperate to get some motion. Nothing changed.

Ida looked at us, moved toward us and, with elbows flying, prodded us out of the way. As we stumbled off, Ida reached over to the client and placed one hand fully open on the base of the sacrum. To my astonishment, the sacrum came rocking and lifting backward. I know and remember all too well how Ida admonished us not to talk of energy. (We were in the full blush of those early magical years at Esalen, the Mecca of the human potential movement.) But on that day, at that moment, Ida connected with the energy of that person on the table and, grabbing onto it, helped his sacrum. There is no way that just physical touch could have provided for that movement. Ida had the connection. She was trying to get us to experience force in a fundamental, physically dense fashion. On that day, I knew Ida was trying to get us by with the basics.

Another memorable day with Ida for me was when a group of Stanford psychiatrists came to Esalen to

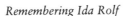

check out what we were doing. All of Esalen showed its stuff (although we did hold back some of our more "out there" Esalen techniques). The Stanford people weren't all that convinced by what we were showing—Gestalt, group dynamics, Rolfing. After the meeting, Ida called me aside and invited me to go along with her to her room. (I think I also had some shoulder pain that needed to be looked at.) Ida and I sat and chatted about the work. She told me that Rolfing had developed a bit at a time; she really had no full idea about it to begin with. It started and then, she said (and I remember my emotion at hearing her), information was coming to her from a deeper, cosmic connection. It was coming to her and through her. I grapple with my memory for the exact words, and while I can't find them, I know that this was the sense of the communication. I had never before heard Ida say this; I felt it to be a special sharing and never told anyone. I wonder even now about this.

There are other Ida-isms and stories to tell, for example, how Ida never really graduated any of us boys to the stature of men. That included some pretty prominent, even world-famous "boys" at that time.

Hector Prestera

One last story: One day Ida came up to my house on the hill above Santa Lucia in Big Sur. I think it was the last time I saw her. We sat outside, looking over the beautiful Big Sur coastline, and Ida explained to me about the great fascial planes and muscular plates in the body and that these could be moved and shifted. She ended by saying I didn't know about that yet—and she was right. I have thought about this through the years and am still trying to learn.

Al Drucker

"Don't Weary of Well-Doing"
Remembrances of a Well-Doer Who Never Wearied

This is my tribute to and recollection of a very great soul, a world-class teacher, and, I make bold to say, a friend—Ida Rolf. But before I speak about her I would like to say a few things about myself and my life during these crucial years before I first encountered Ida. It was the early 1960s. After finding myself in and out of hospitals with severe peptic ulcers, I knew that a drastic change in lifestyle was in the offing. I was then part of a small group of physicists and engineers who had been put together in secret to manage President Eisenhower's super-urgent missile race. We worked night and day to get the different nuclear ballistic missile programs operational in a race with the Soviets. But it became more and more clear to me that I was in the wrong business. It was the new era of the counterculture, and many I knew were dropping out. I went to Israel and Greece to disappear.

In Corfu, at a little café in the hills, I overheard an American couple talk about Esalen. I had been to

Esalen for a weekend earlier that year. Esalen, which at the time was hardly two years old, was rustic and primitive and beautiful and outrageous. I could never quite picture myself living there; it was sort of a Walter Mitty get-away place where the more adventurous, long-buried personas inside me could come to the fore.

For a war-monger busy designing nuclear missiles, I felt strangely at home in this unique place. I will never forget the scene sitting in the Esalen lodge, the only meeting room at that time, and seeing Dick Price, the co-founder of Esalen, running across the deck outside, followed closely by Dennis Murphy, the brother of co-founder Michael Murphy, threateningly holding a length of galvanized pipe over his head. I was told it was Esalen's version of the Cold War.

I sought out Dick afterwards to see if he was OK, and I remember hitting it off with this deeply sensitive and sincere human being. Within a few years he would have counted up more than 500 Rolfings in his body. At the time, he told me about how Ida Rolf had been brought to Esalen from New York by Bernie Gunther to work on Fritz Perls and had saved Fritz's life after he had had two heart attacks. With this background, I introduced myself to this couple in Corfu as one who had tasted a bit of Big Sur life and in many ways found it even more exotic than Greece. My newfound friends showed me an announcement of Esalen's first nine-month residential program, scheduled for the following year. I applied that very day. There were about 200 applicants for fifteen spots. I was accepted.

At that time, Fritz had been donated a newfangled reel-to-reel video recording machine. It was huge and finicky. It almost required a PH.D. to run it. I quickly became Fritz's assistant in charge of videotaping his sessions. Fritz took a liking to me. We spent hours together on his stamp collection and on his art work, much of it done when he lived on the beach in Elath in southern Israel. Noticing that I was a little stoop-shouldered, he told me to see Ida the next time she came to Esalen. Ida was scheduled to do her first Rolfer training program at Esalen. I went to see her to apply for it.

Ida took one look at me and labeled me a near hopeless case. She would not even consider training me until I had been Rolfed. At that time, Ida was planning a scientific research program to be run at a state facility, where she would take obviously misaligned bodies and straighten them out so that they look better even than God had intended them to be. Having been a bookworm all my life and guilty of all the sins of unconscious posture, I was a prime candidate for her before-and-after research program. She insisted that I not get Rolfed except as part of her program. So I had to wait a year. Although Ida spent much time in Big Sur where I was now living, I had to drive a round-trip of 250 miles twice a week to get Rolfed by her and Peter Melchior in Julian Silverman's Rolfing research program at Agnew State Mental Hospital. I leave it to your imagination what it feels like to go to a sprawling state institution and troop through several mental wards to get to the little room where Ida and Peter did their Rolfing.

For me, driving 500 miles a week to get Rolfed was the ultimate sacrifice, but it was worth it. I can't say that I felt so very differently inside, but the body was now functioning like a Rolfed body should, the stoop was gone, there was no more pain, all the joints were well-oiled. I could dance with abandon to the Esalen Thursday night drums, and, most important of all, the before-and-after pictures satisfied Ida's criteria.

She agreed to take me into her next training program, which I believe was in 1970. At the first class meeting I fell totally in love with her. This was a real mensch, a truly human being. Her sensitivity, her compassion, her no-nonsense devotion to her work, her grand sense of humor, her deep wisdom, her easy transitions from her Manhattan lifestyle to the hip

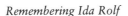

Big Sur culture and from her PH.D. high science to her psychic meta-science, her regal bearing and great personal beauty, her authoritative presence and self-confidence, instantly won me over. This was the teacher I had longed for and searched for in all the great minds and personalities that had come to Esalen during those formative early years.

At the time I was living in a new house in one of the most spectacular places on earth, at the end of a private road in Coastlands, overlooking Pfeiffer Beach and also looking out over an enchanting redwood canyon, a meandering stream, the rocks jutting out into the Pacific Ocean below, wildflowers everywhere. I offered to move out and turn the place over to Ida when she was in Big Sur. She graciously accepted my offer and so, driving her little red VW Beetle with the sunroof open and the fresh rose in her beautiful silver hair reaching for the sun, she would commute twice daily from her Big Sur hideout to her classes at Esalen.

I have many remembrances of Ida during the years that followed. Some of these memories are particularly strongly etched in my consciousness. One time Ida did a training program in the Florida Keys. Some months earlier I had been invited to do Rolfings at a growth center north of Miami. When I got some time free, I went to visit Ida in the Keys. She was most happy to see me and quickly recruited me into the class to lecture on entropy and the inevitable degeneration into chaos of a previously ordered system such as the myofascial tissue, unless new order was brought into the tissues.

I had developed a fairly esoteric spiel on the basic physics of Rolfing and the relationships between gravity, time, entropy, information, and the second law of thermodynamics. Ida always encouraged these kinds of mental exercises, perhaps because they could somehow help to legitimize Rolfing in the prevailing culture. Personally, I was more interested in developing my subtle healing powers and innate knowledge rather than dwelling on intellectual concepts, but I expounded on them for her sake because she liked them, and perhaps because she liked me for presenting them. Funny, today I can't remember a single coherent thought on the subject. Without Ida's interest they have disappeared right back into the vapors.

I had a friend from Esalen named John who was a British Lord and who had inherited a pile of money. He owned a large villa on one of the islands in the Bahamas. John offered to let me stay in his villa any time I liked, all expenses paid, even when he was not there. From the Keys I flew over to John's island to check out his place. It rivaled the legendary Shangri-La. It could not have been more beautiful, with white sandy beaches, crystal clear water, picturesque coral reefs a quarter-mile out, all the yachts, sailboats, snorkel, and fishing equipment one could ever dream of using, large elegantly appointed rooms, native servants, the whole works.

As soon as I got there and looked around and pinched myself a few times to realize that it was real, I got on the phone and called Ida. "Ida, it is so beautiful here. You just have to come and spend some days here, resting and enjoying the island." Quite surprisingly she accepted the invitation, and three days later she and her older son, Dick Demmerle, arrived on the island.

I picked them up by boat and took them to the far side of the island where John had his place. Ida was so relaxed and happy. She was like a little girl. She insisted that we take the boat out to the coral and, while Dick and I dived into the reef exploring the phantasmagoria of colorful sea life below, she stayed in the boat, holding her parasol and very animatedly interested in everything. Whenever we came up for air she would point out a school of fish or a particular coral formation which we should investigate. From above the water inside the boat she couldn't even begin to see one one-hundredth of the splash of colors and huge variety of sea life that we were seeing. But you wouldn't know it from the joy she was having. It is said that beauty is in the eyes of the beholder. Clearly, she saw beauty from her vantage point and was totally and thoroughly delighted.

No sooner did we get to the house (and before she even got unpacked) than she insisted that there was an errant rib in my chest that needed her and Dick's attention. I lay down on the bed in my swim suit. Ida got on one side, Dick on the other, and the rib soon knew who was its master. I howled, begging for relief, but there was no sign of empathy registering on either of their faces, as they resolved to turn this body into a spitting likeness of the pictures in the anatomy book.

But then I noticed something unusual. The feeling was distinctly like being in direct association with a porpoise and a shark. The pain and discomfort were primarily coming from one source. Dick will have to forgive me for saying so, but his Rolfing, at least at that time, was more of a physical process, and he was dutifully moving the rib back into its ideal alignment using physical Rolfing pressure. To me it felt like being attacked by a shark. When Ida took a turn or worked together with Dick on the opposite side of the body, she seemed to energetically coax the offending member to give up its obstreperous behavior and come back into alignment. She somehow Rolfed more energetically and, although it was equally intense, it felt more like lovemaking than pain. With her the experience was more like being at play with a porpoise. She got the work done without a lot of powerful physical pressure.

I spoke to her about this later and she mentioned how you can bring in order by energetic passes alone. After that I saw her many times make passes, slowly circling her hands over a body. When I asked her why she wasn't teaching that, she hushed me and told me to keep it to myself. Somehow the world was not yet ready for that Rolfing refinement. All of the students in her classes have experienced her remarkable facility for looking right through other students standing in the way of her sight, to yell at somebody working at the other end of the room, telling them to stop, that they were in the wrong place in the body they were working on.

How did she manage to see through other people like that? It was a great mystery. But what many Rolfers never knew is the highly developed psychic power she had in other areas, particularly in calming an emotionally distraught model or in making energetic passes over the body to get total pain relief, or in knowing what another person was thinking, making her comments on the subject even before the thoughts had found words in their originator. She frequently said, "There is no psychology; there is only physiology. Align the man and his mind will come into alignment." For her, given her subtle powers, these statements were obviously true. After encountering Ida in a session, many previously intractable aberrations of the mind would quite suddenly disappear.

One time when I was assisting Ida in her class at Esalen, Moshe Feldenkrais dropped in to pay his respects. He was a charming, affable European gentleman with an Israeli, desert-honed toughness and a pixyish playfulness. He clearly had a winning way about him. Feldenkrais held a doctorate of physics from the Sorbonne, had developed a very successful surface-to-surface missile for the Israeli Navy, and had been karate champion of Europe for years. In his later years he had developed his own system of bodywork. His method utilized some brilliant insights into the workings of the mind, making use of the mind's peculiar method of recruiting individual muscle groups to perform their tasks. He tended to pooh-pooh the efficacy of most other systems of bodywork, but he had a deep regard for Ida and the brilliance of her understanding of the organization of the body. So, he felt there were only two systems of bodywork that were worth anything, the Feldenkrais Method and Rolfing.

When I first met Moshe Feldenkrais, at the time

he visited the Rolfing class, I liked him immediately but I also thought this little roly-poly man was not very impressive from a Rolfing point of view. Ida must have felt likewise. Before he could even say much to the class about his latest discoveries, Ida had him take off his outer clothes and get on the table, and she instructed me to Rolf him. On the outside he was like butter; on the inside he was hard as steel. Over the years, it took many sessions to turn his karate-trained psoas into supple living tissue. He was always deeply appreciative of the work and we would spend some high-quality time together.

The only other master that I worked on that had a body like his was Babaji (Baba Hari Das), a very great silent yogi. He had the same availability on the outside but sinews of pure steel within. There also it took me almost fifteen sessions to reach into the deeper layers. Babaji was warm and loving, but totally unidentified with his body. He showed no signs of pain or delight.

Feldenkrais, on the other hand, was a big teddy bear, responding to every move, making luscious sounds, commenting on every brain-signal pathway that was being affected or redirected by the work. He thoroughly enjoyed himself in the Rolfing process. It was a great research project for him with opportunities to directly experience new discoveries of bodily connections. He would get off the table after a particularly effective move and show me on my body how he would have done it using a very different but frequently equally effective method of manipulation. He just loved Ida and always spoke highly of her.

Another interesting person I had a chance to work on was Zalman Schachter, a well-known Chassidic rabbi with something of a hippie following. He had attended one of our Rolfing demos during the week he was leading a group at Esalen, and he was very impressed. He wanted to experience the work firsthand himself. When during the first hour I worked on his chest, he started to cry out with delight, "You're making me kosher! You're making me kosher!" Later he explained that for orthodox Jews, the meat of an animal could not be eaten if the flesh sticks to the bones. You have to be able to pass your hand between the innermost fascial layer and easily separate it from the ribs underneath for the animal to be kosher. Well, before the first Rolfing hour, he considered himself *treif,* ritually unclean. But the Rolfing was a great sacrament that made him kosher, at last. Later in the session, his joy knew no bounds. When I was working on his pelvis he yelled out, "O, get him! Get him! Get that *dibbuk!*" He felt he had a demon living in his pelvis and now mercifully I was expunging that dibbuk forever. Zalman was such a joy to

Rolf I didn't ever want to stop and finish the session.

A few years after I had been trained by Ida there was a big movement at Esalen and on the Big Sur coast in general to go study with an exceptional Chilean master, a disciple of Gurdjieff and an accomplished yogi and martial arts expert whose name was Oscar Ichazo. Ram Dass, whom most of us knew as Dick Alpert, and who was no stranger to the Big Sur coast, and Claudio Naranjo, a Chilean psychiatrist and meditation teacher who led workshops at Esalen, came back from a trip to Arica, Chile, and spoke glowingly of Ichazo and his school. More than fifty people from Big Sur decided to go to Chile and take the Arica training. I planned to be among them. But when I told Ida of my plans, she nixed them. "You stay here and become a good Rolfer before you go off to do anything else. Do this work for five years; then it will be part of you and you can go off and study anything you like without your hands forgetting how to Rolf." I stayed and launched into a bevy of Rolfings. Many days I would do as many as seven Rolfings, one after the other. My hands developed their own innate knowing. I was becoming a Rolfer.

One day a new teacher came quite by chance to visit Esalen. It was Professor Worseley from Oxford, England, where he had a College of Chinese Medicine. I asked Ida if I could go to England and study acupuncture with Dr. Worseley. This time she had no strong objection. I went to England and spread the news of this wonderful new system of bodywork, called Structural Integration, and worked my way through the acupuncture program doing Rolfings.

I should like to mention something about our Wednesday evening Rolfing demos at Esalen during the early days. At that time not many Rolfers had been trained but, nevertheless, many seminarians coming to Esalen had had some Rolfings. We knew most of the Rolfers and their idiosyncrasies. Some had missed, let's say, the second hour in the class or never really gotten it, but were very expert in the third hour, for example. In these demos a couple of us Rolfers, such as Ed Maupin and myself, would invite anyone in the audience to come up, take off their clothes, and let us guess if they had been Rolfed and how many sessions they had had. It was amazing in those early days before a lot of other deep bodywork had been developed or had become popularly known how clearly the Rolfing left a signature on the body. We could almost always tell if the person had been Rolfed or not. Three-quarters of the time we could even tell within one or two hours how many sessions they had had. And about a third of the time we would tell them who their Rolfer had been, when we could see a particular hour had been missed or not very thoroughly done but a later hour clearly showed up. It was magic. We continuously surprised ourselves at the accuracy of our guesses. It made a powerful impression on people and sharpened their seeing. After we demonstrated a first hour, most of the people in the room could clearly see the effects of the session, and eagerly signed up to get the work.

About once a month or sometimes every other month, usually on a Saturday, the Rolfers in the area would get together at Esalen and we would have the Rolf-monster. With the aid of a little mushroom, we would work on each other, five or six Rolfers working at once on one body. It was intense, really intense. You can imagine what it would be like to get a seventh hour with several pairs of hands working on and inside your head. It was surprising that we all survived these meetings without broken bones or psychotic breakdowns. Perhaps it was the wonderful camaraderie and trust we felt towards each other and the fear of Ida's fury if anything untoward happened and she found out. In fact, these Rolf-monster meetings for the most part turned out to be wonderful; it was a great way to get our bodies worked on and to share new discoveries.

During her last years, during the time when Ida was suffering from cancer, I had left Esalen and gone to India to live at Sai Baba's ashram. There I taught at the university and immersed myself in spiritual studies. Both the Rolfing and acupuncture fell by the wayside. I might have dropped doing Rolfing, but I certainly didn't drop Ida. Although in the years after having been trained by Ida, I had studied with many other great teachers and learned a number of other powerful healing systems, Ida was my principal teacher, the one I most revered and whom I followed before I came to Baba, who is my *sadguru,* my ultimate spiritual teacher.

I wrote to Ida periodically and shared some of the deeper experiences I was having in India. I wrote to her of Baba and of the great saints of India, particularly the nondualists like Ramana Maharshi and Nisargadatta, and the great devotees of God, like Ramakrishna, the depth of whose inner passion for truth had touched me deeply. I always felt strongly connected with her in these letters, knowing that she would be deeply interested. Occasionally I heard back from her. Clearly she had a rich inner life, because she showed a profound understanding of spiritual philosophy and spiritual practice. At a time when she must have been suffering terribly, she let me know how happy she was to receive my letters and touch in on these great ancient teachings of the Vedanta, which Aldous Huxley called the perennial wisdom of the East.

When I published a version of the *Bhagavad Gita,* based on a series of discourses given by Sai Baba, she had her attendants read portions to her and would go off into periods of reverie. Baba has said that the true meaning of enjoy is to "end in joy," to be fully at peace at the moment of transition from this corporeal home to the freedom beyond. I was in India when Ida died. Somehow I knew that she was in joy, having lived a rich life of service to mankind, never wearying of well-doing.

So now, on your 100th birthday, we salute you and offer our sacred *pranams* to you, our dear older sister. You have given so much to so many and shared the goodness of your immense heart with all the generations yet to come. We love you, sweet Ida. Happy Happy Birthday! We all celebrate your birth and our treasure of warm memories recalling the time when you graced us by your presence among us.

Sharon Wheeler-Hancoff

Fritz Perls convinced me to get Rolfed. We were walking up from the baths at Esalen when he stopped at the bench near the top of the hill and remarked that before Rolfing he had had to stop there and rest-twenty minutes before he could make it to the lodge. After Rolfing he didn't have to stop anymore. I was a massage practitioner at Esalen, so I knew how deep you had to push to hurt someone. I had observed bruises from Rolfing and had not seen any changes in my friends who had been Rolfed. I thought Rolfing was crazy.

I asked Fritz, "Is Rolfing really any good for you?" He said, "Let me put it this way. . . ." If he forgot anything at his house at the start of the day (cigarettes, telephone book, etc.), it used to stay forgotten. He had just enough energy to make it from his house to the lodge for breakfast—to his morning group—to lunch and the baths for the afternoon—to dinner—his group—and back to his house again. After Rolfing, he could go anywhere he liked. I thought that over and decided that if Fritz could survive Rolfing, I could too. So I became the first person Jan Sultan Rolfed after class, something neither of us has forgotten, Jan assures me.

The first time I met Ida Rolf was about 1967, at a Los Angeles class. She suggested we go into the kitchen and have some tea. I was embarrassed to confess I had no idea how to make tea. So she made it the English way. I also didn't have a whole lot to say—being about twenty years old. I remember she was very kind to me and seemed happy to get away from her class for a while.

Sometime during the six-week period of the class, it occurred to me that I might be able to do this work. Toward the end of the class I gathered my courage and spoke with Dr. Rolf, asking her if she would consider training me. She looked me over and thought about it for so long I was sure she was thinking of something devastating to say to turn me down. She had just announced she wasn't going to train any more women or anyone under 140 pounds and no more non-professionals. Then she turned to Rosemary and said, "I'll train her—put her in the next class." I was relieved and happy and amazed.

The next class was two weeks away. Since everyone had to read five anatomy books and write a paper, I assumed she expected the same from me—in two weeks. I began to study. I had to look up every third term to understand any of the book, and had read two-thirds of the anatomy book in order to get through the first few pages. At this rate, I knew I wasn't going to make it, and, down at heart, I confessed to Dr. Rolf that I didn't think I was going to get the reading done and write a paper in time for the next class. She eyed me with some disbelief and told me she didn't expect me to do it. In fact, she didn't want me to know any anatomy. She didn't know any anatomy when she started and only learned it later to be able to talk to people. She told me I didn't need it to learn how to Rolf. In fact, whenever I looked at an anatomy book in class, she made me put it down.

Both of my classes were held in Jan Breuer's River House in Big Sur. I remember some well-educated participants: Hector Prestera, M.D., an internist and cardiologist; Fritz Smith, D.O.; Al Drucker, an aerospace engineer; Bill Williams, PH.D., a psychologist; Owen James, a silver flute player; and me. I remember Dr. Rolf making a remark about her "artistic experiments." My guess is that I was one of them.

During my practitioner class, Dr. Rolf took some delight in using me to show up the large men. She would tap them on the shoulder and tell them to sit down. Then she would tell me to get in there and show them how to do it. Al Drucker, who had studied his anatomy so that he knew it better than the doctors, got so exasperated with my ability he began calling me the "idiot savant" of Rolfing. A year or so later, he asked her why she had picked me. She told him it was because I saw bodies the same way she did.

Another Al Drucker tidbit: Rosemary tells me that in a previous class Al had told her the following joke: What is the difference between a professional and an amateur? An amateur says "whoops" when he makes a mistake; a professional says "there." So when I slipped off a woman's third-hour line on her leg and said "whoops," Dr. Rolf had the perfect line, which was, "My dear, never say, 'whoops,' always say, 'there!'"

She was unfailingly kind to me. She never raised her voice or put me down. She didn't hesitate to do either with other people. Early in my practitioner class, I was doing a third hour on my model when she tapped me on the shoulder and said, "I can see you know what you're doing. You look tired. Go sit down and I'll finish this up for you." I sat there trying not to cry. When the model left, she said to me, "You really wanted to finish that, didn't you?" I nodded yes. She said, "Well, next time, I'll let you."

She taught me differently from the other students in class. She would have me feel an area. Then either

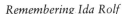

she would work on it or she would put her hands on mine and work through my hands and then have me feel it again. She would stop me and ask me where I was going next. Once when I was working on a leg—one arm on the hip and a fist near the knee—she stopped me and asked me where I was working. I pointed to a place between my points of contact, thinking how impossible an answer it was as I wasn't touching in that place. She nodded and said, "That's right."

She had a brilliant mind and remains the only person I heard speak who knew where she was in the flow of time. I can still read what she wrote and whole new vistas open up for me. I have not seen her equal as a practitioner either (my apologies to various egos). She had an intolerance for bad Rolfing and no patience for "chit-chat."

She had the disconcerting habit of telling people she thought they were the best of her students. I suspect this got them quite devoted and willing to work for Rolfing that much harder. Several people I know were told they were the best (and some probably still believe it). Ah, well—politics. I know she was very concerned that Rolfing should survive her death and she sacrificed a tremendous amount of personal time and money as well as her respected status as a biochemist to further this work. She would always have VIPs in class to be Rolfed. These were people who, if they talked about the benefits of her work, she hoped would help to shortcut the time it takes for recognition.

A big part of her teaching was in telling stories about people's sessions. These stories were phrased in plain, kind of homey language. I remember one story about a man who came in complaining of pain in his neck. She looked at him and told him that in her opinion his neck was fine, the trouble was in his legs. They had this conversation a few times—he saying neck, she working on his legs. Finally, during a leg session, he started crying, "The ropes! Your hands feel just like the ropes on my legs." The history was that he had been kidnapped at five years old; his legs were tied up and he was left in a garden shed for many hours until his family found him.

Dr. Rolf would teach us to recognize the age at which a trauma occurred, describing ten-year-old legs, a three-year-old arm still persisting in the adult. One story I still think about was when she stopped Rolfing a model in class and asked him to tell her about the bicycle accident he had had when he was five years old. And he did! I can see the five-year-old—but the *bicycle*?

Another magic moment was when a Rolfer brought in a woman on whom he had done ten sessions, for critique and suggestions. The client stood there for a few short seconds; then Dr. Rolf said, "You're Rolfing her in a room that is too small." And yes—he was Rolfing her in an attic room with low ceilings.

It was 1979—the Philadelphia advanced class. Ida was working on Francis Wenger (who won't mind my telling this story). I had the habit of getting close and watching carefully whenever she would work. To my great admiration and awe, I saw her open up the right pulmonary artery. I could see that Francis was feeling the new circulatory pattern and that it was tickling in his lungs. He was trying not to laugh about it. So I said quietly to him, "Tickles, doesn't it?" He nodded and smiled. Dr. Rolf, who was now working on his legs, looked up and asked, "What tickles?" I felt silly explaining, but told her that because she had just opened his right pulmonary artery the new circulation was tickling inside like champagne bubbles. Francis laughed and agreed. Dr. Rolf said nothing for a few minutes and continued working a little on his legs. Then she gave me a long look and said, "You know, a hundred years ago, they would have burned you."

You may have noticed that each and every Rolfer has a different "feel." Having seen and felt Dr. Rolf, I should try to describe how she worked:

Because of her ability to see, she seemed to select

the most key areas with major historical trauma and extreme sensation levels. She was able to reach right in and take firm hold of the tissue involved. She was dead-on accurate. In doing so, the sensation level was often beyond complaining about. The work brought the historic memory to the surface very rapidly for me. And, of course, once the memory began to un-roll, the sensation level would lessen to so little as to be beneath further notice. I both dreaded seeing her coming and simultaneously rejoiced because I knew she would resolve the problem.

She addressed tissue with a wide variety of pres-sures and movements to achieve her functional goals. Long sweeping strokes on tissue she called "ironing" (also because this tends to produce burning). She would use the tips of straight fingers and bring her wrists down—she called this "shoveling." She would flip tissue back and forth, large areas with an elbow or forearm, smaller areas with fingers or knuckles. She called this "playing the guitar" or "strumming." And much, much more.

She spoke of tissue having a direction and said that if you pushed on it, it would give in the "right di-rection." She almost always used two points of con-tact, and almost always asked for movement. I remember the phrase, "take it where it belongs and call for movement."

She never did the same session the same way twice, and though she held the rest of us to one hour, upon occasion she would work up to three hours on a session. I have seen her work with internal organs and bones if they were in trouble. She also related to each student differently and consistently. She was a wonderfully diverse teacher. She knew how difficult it was for students and had some sayings both teasing and teaching. "Where you think it is, it ain't." "If at first you don't succeed—get the hell out." And, "the only rule in Rolfing is that there are no rules." I also remember her comment that all of the talk about fascia, theories about how Rolfing worked, were only theories. The only thing we can say for certain, she said, is that if you push on it, it will move.

As I look at all the Rolfers and teachers she trained, I see that most of them favor one or two ways of working on tissue. Everyone seems to have picked up what they can understand and what works for them. To get closer to the whole picture of what Ida Rolf really did, I think it would be best to study with as many different people as possible.

I keep as a guiding principle from her a statement she really did mean: "The goal of Rolfing is nothing less than the integration of the field of the body with the field of the earth."

Beverly Silverman

I can remember Diane W. showing off the marks on her rib cage as if they were medals. This was 1968 at Esalen Institute in Big Sur, California. I remember thinking that it was bizarre, and a little perverse, to have someone stick their fingers in your body and do whatever it was, as she tried to explain, that a Rolfer does. I definitely wasn't interested in submitting myself to something obviously weird.

But when I met Ida, I was so impressed with the life force that seemed to radiate from her eyes. She seemed more alive than all of the younger people around her and I wanted some of that. She wasn't very tall, around 5'6", and she was square and built like a tank. Whenever I saw her, she almost always had a fresh flower in her very white hair. . . . But I still wasn't convinced that Rolfing was safe.

It was about a year later that Stan Johnson, a medical doctor who was in the Rolfing training, called me and asked if I would be interested in being his model. I said YES! I was still intrigued by what I

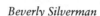

heard about this old lady and what she was doing. Also, because Stan was a doctor, I figured he at least would know where *not* to put his fingers.

I was a timid and dependent type at this stage in my life. Although I had no "serious" problems, I was pretty rigid in my randomness. I had poor circulation and a poor connection in my articulations—my energy had trouble passing from my trunk to my legs.

Needless to say, but I will anyway, the Rolfing changed my life—as it has for so many others. The changes that I felt were more energetic than structural at first. Before the Rolfing, I always felt as if I were behind myself with my willpower pushing my body to operate—to move. With the Rolfing I began to enjoy moving and to feel a coherence between my head and my body. By the eighth session I decided that I had to know more about this method that was having so much effect on me. I said out loud that I wanted to learn Rolfing—Ida said out louder—NO! I asked why and she said that I was too small. (I can't swear if she said after that, or if I just *thought* she said, that I was a woman with small children and should stay home and care for my family.) I said I was small but had strong hands. She said NO! At the time she was also looking for people to train to work with children. I said that I could work on children. She said NO! She said children were even harder to work on than grown-ups.

But the Rolfing had done its job on me and I refused to take her no's! as a definite response. I returned to the university to prepare myself with classes in anatomy and physiology. I continued to see Ida because I was often at Esalen and my husband at the time was involved in a research project with Valerie Hunt on the effects of Rolfing. So at every opportunity I would say that I wanted to be a Rolfer, and as many times as I would say it in front of her, as many times she would say NO!

Then one day I received a telephone call from Rosemary Feitis saying that there was a place in the next training for an auditor, and would I be interested—she had to be kidding! That was the summer of 1970.

I loved the training. I audited in the River House in Big Sur, about twenty-five miles up the road from where we (family) were staying at Esalen. I can't remember everyone who was in the class, but I do remember that we had a great time. Each morning on the ride up I had butterflies in my stomach. It was the beginning of an exciting day. I remember the smell of the air like a favorite perfume—a mix of salt, eucalyptus, and damp earth being warmed by the sun. What a fragrance. It was also the time of Fritz Perls and Will Schutz, Steely Dan and The Stones, in the here-and-now era.

In the auditing stage, we were not allowed to touch. Just look—and look—and look—until we finally saw. Because it was a very tiring (and I have to admit, sometimes boring) way to learn, Ida was asked a lot why she set up the auditing in that way. She would give one of her sighs, roll her eyes, and then say that she hadn't found a better way to change people's way of looking and seeing differently. She was trying to teach us to see things in relationship (among other things) and not the linear way that we had been taught. You look, you look, you look, until finally . . . you can *see*.

The morning was the lecture, always starting with: What is Rolfing? What is the first hour?, etc. No matter how many times she asked the same questions there were always new things to learn.

Then "coffee break." Coffee break was important. Ida took her coffee with heavy cream (she was into animal protein) and she loved her cakes. Since I was one of the few women in the class, I was the coffee maker. Ida came from the old school where "it's the woman's job, etc." In the beginning that didn't bother me because that's where I came from too, but as the Rolfing continued to change my body and therefore my head, I realized that Ida was a bit of a misogynist. Oh, well, no one is perfect.

I loved the classes. Mac, a rehabilitation medicine

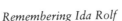

Remembering Ida Rolf

M.D., was an auditor at the same time that I was. It was fun to watch his face as Ida with her magic fingers and Rolfing principles challenged his preconceived notions about the body and how it works. I was lucky because I didn't have too many preconceived notions—in fact I don't think I had many notions at all at that time in my life. I was a slate upon which the principles of Rolfing were being etched (or so I'd like to think). I was learning how to see—I was learning how to think—I was learning how to speak—I was learning how to walk—I was learning how to feel—using my body as a reference.

I responded to her allegory that working with the fascia is like the starched curtains that were dried on a wooden curtain frame with needles. You start in one corner, then go to another, and as you tug one place you see the effect in another. (My mother had one of those things when I was little and I was intrigued by the process.) I also responded to the metaphor of cleaning off the gunk. It was a very visual image and has served me well when I haven't known what to do next in a session.

At the end of the auditing class, Rosemary came over and asked if I wanted to be in the practitioner class. There was not time for a pause between her question and my response. Then Rosemary added, "Ida said don't think this means that you're going to be a Rolfer. . . ." She sure knew how to keep a girl on her toes.

The next class was to be in San Diego in the fall (it was then summer 1970), and when I started to think out loud how I was going to organize my personal life and my kids so that I could go, Ida heard! "Oh, no," she said, "you can't come if you have to uproot your kids. You'll have to wait until next summer." So . . . I waited.

This time the training was in the Joe Adams house, again in Big Sur. Boulder wasn't yet in the picture. We used to walk around in the exaggerated "elbows out, lumbars back" position—we were trying to discover the new way to walk! Also, as we all know who have gone through the Rolfing training, it is a very intense time. Being Rolfed twice a week is already intense. Add to that being Rolfed by someone who is in the process of learning and it can be explosive. We sure did have a lot of explosive learning experiences!

If you were looking for compliments, it wasn't around Ida that you would find them. The closest that I came to a *gentillesse* was as I was doing a session and was inching my way up the body because I was so afraid of missing something important. Ida, who was watching, asked if I knew the rhyme of the bedbug. When I said no, I heard for the first time:

Butterflies fly on wings of gold,
Fireflies fly on flame,
Bedbugs have no wings at all,
But they get there just the same.

I think that was an Ida compliment.

I didn't find Ida "warm and caring" like the projections one could have on her physical person. Fortunately I wasn't looking for a grandmother so I wasn't disappointed. I did find her honest, perceptive, intelligent . . . and a real Zen Master.

It has been twenty-five years this year since I've been Rolfing and I can tell you that I'm still working and living with the Rolfing principles. I still find the work new and exciting, and I still depend on the recipe when I don't know what to do next.

Thank you, Ida.

Annie Duggan
A Few Memories That Have Stayed With Me

I remember the first time I met Ida. My husband at the time, Ron McComb, was hired to help with illustrations for the book Ida was writing. We went into a class she was teaching at Kairos in Rancho Santa Fe, California. Giovanna D'Angelo was in the back of the room taking photographs of the models. Nothing was coming out on the Polaroids. Giovanna came out of the room and said to Ida, "Stop it, Ida, we can't get any images on the photographs, you have to stop blocking it." Giovanna went back in and we proceeded to take photographs without any trouble.

As I paid attention to the class, I was intrigued and fascinated. Ida was talking with one of the models and explaining to the students in the class about what she was seeing in his structure. Then someone blocked her line of vision and she said, "I can see through furniture, but I cannot see through another person." We all laughed, but later on, in my experience with Ida, this statement proved to be very true.

As I got to know Ida and Rosemary Feitis, who at

that time was Ida's right hand, they were a delight to watch. They sparred in good humor with each other, but it was clear there was real caring and respect between them. One day Rosemary, Ida, and I went to the movies to see *The Sound of Music,* Ida's favorite movie at the time. Coming out of the movie theater after the show we were waiting for Rosemary. Ida looked up and saw a poster of the movie. She proceeded to get on her toes, and while doing a little whirl she sang the theme. She looked so carefree and young.

After Rancho Santa Fe we continued to stay with Ida as she moved to her next class in Big Sur. I used to sometimes bring tea to her in the afternoons after her nap. It was one afternoon as she was waking up that we started to talk about age. The most disconcerting thing to her was that in her mind her image of herself was that she was still about thirty years old.

But, when she looked in the mirror, she was shocked to see this old person looking back at her. Since that conversation twenty-five years ago, I now know what she meant. With love and respect.

Ron McComb

When I met Dr. Rolf, one of the first things she said to me was, "Tell me, young man, you look like you might know how the shoulder girdle fits on the body ... I don't." My reaction was, "Gee, I just got here." It wasn't until years later that Peter Melchior told me her comment about the shoulder girdle was my assignment, and that, as far as he knew, almost everyone who knew her then had an assignment. Mine was also to make photographs as illustrations in her forthcoming book.

Before I left that first meeting, she said that she couldn't stand to have anyone leave her presence in as much back pain as I was in. She sat me down and placed one of her trusty knuckles in my back for about ten seconds and then said that should hold me until January when I could begin my first ten sessions as a class model. When I stood up it felt as if she had lifted 300 pounds off my back. A week later, while standing in the shower, I suddenly felt as though I were standing in an earthquake. Every part of my body rearranged itself and I suddenly felt taller, more centered, out of pain, and clearer than I could remember ever feeling. Her prophecy proved true; my body didn't begin to collapse into its old self again until about three days before the January class started.

I was given a room next to the classroom to set up the photo area. I spent the day before the class setting up, checking the lighting, and doing test exposures to make sure everything would go without a hitch the next morning. When I was done I closed the door and locked it. The next morning I went in to begin shooting pictures. I pulled the first exposure. It was blank, white, which meant that it had been overexposed. I tried again. No image. This time it was black, which meant it had not been exposed. I tried again, with the same result. Even though I had successfully used the same film pack in the camera for test exposures the night before, I thought something must have happened to it.

Time was wasting, so I hurriedly changed to a new film pack. The first exposure was still blank. I knew this camera so well I could practically build one from scratch and I checked it thoroughly, thinking perhaps the shutter was sticking. It worked perfectly. Giovanna D'Angelo was standing nearby listening to Ida hold forth in the classroom. Sensing my frustration, she asked me what was going on. After hearing my complaint she said, "I think I know what's wrong." She went into the classroom and interrupted Dr. Rolf: "Ida, you've got to turn it off. Ron can't get a picture in here." The next shot was perfect. I had done nothing between the previous failure and the one following Giovanna's intervention. As if Dr. Rolf's intervention in my back hadn't been convincing enough, at this point I was made deeply aware that I was involved in something more than a mere exchange of skills.

Somewhere around the fourth or fifth session, I sat up in bed around 4 A.M. out of a dream that led me to say to myself, "I could do this work." Then I went back to sleep. The next morning while I was puttering around with the camera stuff, I noticed that Rosemary seemed to be watching me closely. Suddenly she said, "You're different this morning." I said something like, "Well, I'm being Rolfed." She said, "That's not it." After studying me a few moments longer she said, "You decided to become a Rolfer, didn't you?" Is this sensitivity or what? No wonder she and Ida were so close. In fact I had almost forgotten my statement to myself earlier that same morning. I said something to the effect that it had occurred to me, and kept on working while she went into the classroom where Ida was having her morning tea.

When Rosemary returned she offhandedly said that Ida wanted to see me. I went in to where Ida was and she asked me to sit down. Those who've never met Dr. Rolf will have a hard time imagining how such a little old grandma could suddenly seem eight feet tall while merely sitting having tea. In this imperious persona she looked down at me and said, "Rosemary tells me you want to be a Rolfer." "The thought occurred to me, yes." "Well, I must tell you that my reaction is a final and definite no." Now, even though I might not have seriously entertained the possibility before, this stance forced me to ask, "Why?" "Because you have a soft structure . . . this is hard work that will break down a body as soft as yours and I'll not be responsible for the breakdown of your body." "It is my body, I'm responsible for it." "Hmmmmph . . . well, you realize that if you were ever to become a Rolfer you would have to work on a higher table than most of us because of the problem in your back." "No problem, I'm also a competent carpenter, I can make a table to whatever height I need." "Hummmmph . . . OK then, you've got to realize that when you become a Rolfer you will have to settle down with your new family . . . you can't travel around like Rosemary and I do." So in three sentences I went from no possibility to certainty. Those who complain of Ida's toughness simply are mistaken. I never received anything but the utmost consideration and caring from Ida P. Rolf. In many ways she could be immovable, and nearly as often it would seem to be a front that was meant to be challenged.

The class progressed from one minor miracle to another until a miracle of major consideration occurred. Dr. Rolf's model was a man who had been in an auto accident that created a discontinuity in his spinal nerve at around T3. He had use of his arms but nothing lower down in his body. At one point when she was working on his foot his whole leg jerked so violently that his foot left Ida's hands. Then at the end of his tenth session, Dr. Rolf had him sit unassisted on a backless Rolfing bench. It took me years to realize that she was demonstrating that the passive organ of form was capable of maintaining balance on its own in gravity, without muscular activity.

At one point, Mac MacDonald was working on my back while I was sitting on the floor. Dr. Rolf was looking away from where we were, while telling Mac to work a little further to the left with his right hand. We both commented that she was looking away and Mac said that there was also a bed between her and his hands. Later on that same day I was sitting next to her hoping to get some idea of how she saw. A Rolfer stepped between her and what she was looking at and she said: "Hal! Get out of the way. I can see through beds but not through people."

I began to understand that for Ida, accurate perception was an overriding consideration not only in Rolfing but in life itself. She discovered the principles of Rolfing by struggling to see into the as yet unknown possibilities for easing human misery.

At one point when Ida and I were sitting out on the balcony watching the sunset, I mentioned that I had had déjà vu experiences and asked her if she felt we had all done this before. She said certainly but that this time we had to make it a permanent fixture in the culture so we wouldn't have to do it all over again.

During this time, our newborn daughter stopped eating and soon began to dehydrate. We rushed her to the hospital. Here I saw that even in the area of their greatest expertise, that of saving lives, allopaths are lacking in sensitivity and often in common sense. I had to intervene in their obsessive fixation on testing, which required sticking needles into her tiny body over and over again. When we returned to Esalen from the hospital, we asked Dr. Rolf to work on her. She placed Siobhan on the bed and said, "Ron, would you get me some water from the kitchen, and Annie, would you get me a towel from the bathroom." By the time we returned she had finished her task. Then a week or so later we asked her to work on Siobhan again. Again she asked me to get water and Annie to get a towel. While I was drawing water, I understood what was happening and hurried back into the room just as Dr. Rolf finished. I couldn't believe we'd fallen for the same trick twice. I noticed later on that Siobhan seemed to be able to sit up straight, even at only a few weeks old.

I did get to see Dr. Rolf work on Siobhan about a year or so later when we were all gathered at Esalen for Dr. Rolf's birthday. Siobhan had just begun to walk. Dr. Rolf and I were sitting together on the deck watching her. I commented that Siobhan was walking with her legs stiff like Frankenstein. At about this moment Siobhan got close enough for Ida to reach out and scoop her up into her lap. She worked on her legs for a few seconds and set her back down again. Siobhan walked away using her knees. She stopped, turned, and gave Ida the most incredulous look, then spent the rest of the day dancing.

At Esalen, watching a movie of Master Cheng demonstrating the t'ai chi form, Ida observed that every stable population seemed to evolve to a point where their proportions were all very much alike. Some of the populations that had long unbroken cultural development had evolved forms of structural intervention that matched their proportions. She pointed out that the proportions of Asiatic people, and especially the Chinese, seemed to be based on the sphere. It would be only natural, therefore, for them to develop something like t'ai chi, which was like a rolling sphere. Caucasian proportions seemed to be more ovoid, which created a vertical reference to the gravitational field. She went on to point out that northern Indian people seemed to have proportions that favored yoga. She also said that most of them were vegetarians going back hundreds of generations, which made their deep tissues more flexible than those in cultures inhabited by populations of meat and fat eaters.

Richard Price, co-founder and a guiding light of Esalen, had the reputation of probably having been Rolfed more times than nearly any person alive. He insisted on a Rolfer on staff so he could get a session whenever he wanted one. One day Dr. Rolf and I were watching him crossing the lawn. Dr. Rolf said, "That man's stress is no longer in his body." I'm still working on that one.

In 1976 I signed up for what turned out to be one of Dr. Rolf's last advanced classes. Several episodes stand out. Somewhere near the beginning of the class, during a moment when I felt that no one but she and I were listening, I quietly said something like, "It seems that a major obstacle to learning Rolfing is the opinions we have about what we're seeing, and so I've struggled to reveal my ignorance so that you might see what I need to know." She said rather loudly, "Well, you've certainly done that all right." In this frame of reference I asked her for a definition of sleeve and core. After a long consideration she said, "Core is whatever you can't live without."

Another exchange occurred when I asked her if there were any guidelines to somatotypes. She said, "One could determine somatotype by asking a person, 'How do you feel?' If you were to ask an ectomorph, you would most likely hear them begin by saying, 'Well, I *think* I feel . . .' If you were to ask a mesomorph, you would likely hear a description of their physical reality with words like strength, weakness, pain, tiredness, etc. If you were to ask an endomorph, you had better be prepared to sit down for a long discussion of emotional well-being." She went on to say that she never saw a good psychic that wasn't an endomorph.

During this class, Ida was rather physically weak so she decided to focus on working on babies. As it happened I was staying with friends in NYC who had a six-month-old baby girl who had also been stuck with needles to save her life as a newborn. This child had never been able to sit up or crawl. After a few minutes sitting on Ida's lap screaming while Ida worked on her, she got down and crawled across the bed. Then she sat up and looked at Ida with that same incredulous look, crawled back across the bed, back into Ida's lap for more work.

Sometime near the end of the class, it came time for Dr. Rolf to put her hands on me. Her weakness determined that she would have to select the key in my body that would be the most beneficial with the least amount of effort on her part. She placed her fingers on the left anterior aspect of my atlas and asked me to turn my head to the right. The results of this simple movement were so profound that I left the class determined to gain an understanding of what she could only point toward in this final gesture she made in my life.

Hal Milton

In going through my training with Ida in 1970, she often chided me to go deeper or to change direction as I worked. I would get exasperated as she continued to challenge me, yet she always knew how to stretch me beyond my limitations. In answer to my frustration, Ida would say, "Whom God loveth, He chasteneth."

Michael Salveson

It has been seventeen years since Dr. Rolf's death, and the memories I have of her are so entwined in the unfolding of my own life, in which she has played such a large part, that I give up all hope of presenting anything but my very personal view of her. Events and people swirled around her in a maelstrom of activity, which she orchestrated for the accomplishment of her overarching ambition: the development of Rolfing. I was always struck by the perseverance and sometimes seeming ruthlessness with which she pursued her vision. As I became more deeply involved with her, one of the many assisting her in her work, I was always cautious around her, lest I be sucked into the maelstrom and my life subsumed to her purposes.

The energy around Ida was immense. Her capacity for work and sustained concentration was at a level I had never encountered. Most importantly, I was struck by her intelligence and her unique abilities as a healer. I knew when I met her that she was a real teacher, that I was fortunate indeed to be in her presence, and that it was not likely that I would meet many others of her quality.

I was Ida's assistant in a training class she was teaching in Big Sur during the summer of 1973. We were working to develop her ideas of fascia, and she had asked that I deliver a few morning lectures on fascial anatomy. I spent my evenings studying texts, searching for useful descriptions of fascial structures to be presented in my few morning lectures. Without exception, I would begin my carefully structured presentation and Ida would systematically interrupt, disrupting the intellectual order I had so laboriously built into my talks. I was at a loss, until she said to me, "That's all very nice, Michael, but what is essential is not these pictures you paint from the details in books but the living tissue under your hands. It is clear perception that will ultimately make you a good Rolfer." I realized she had been interrupting me in order to push me and the class into a direct experience of the flesh with which we were working, and out of our intellectually comfortable images. Her lesson came crashing home and I developed an abiding respect for her teaching skills. She had always said, "Leave your *amour-propre* at the door."

Esalen had generously provided Ida a small house on the coast of Big Sur in which to teach during the summers. The large central room served as a classroom and she lived in the rest of the house. Each morning we would assemble, chairs in a circle, at one end of the large room, next to the windows looking out through the Monterey pines onto the Pacific ocean. Ida sat in a large wooden rocking chair for the morning lecture.

I loved her morning lectures. I loved the careful way she used words. The almost Victorian respect she had for language contrasted sharply with the vernacular of the alternative culture she drew many of her students from. As she developed her topic for the morning, she would punctuate her lecture with stories and anecdotes that provided a sort of moral education. With the tea breaks and the students working in the garden, fixing things around the house, the atmosphere was decidedly domestic, a sharp contrast to the anonymity of a university classroom.

She always wore her hair up on her head, usually with a flower. It was her view that hair was heavy and if it was long, it pulled on the back of the head, creating strain in the cervical spine. Therefore, it should be worn on the top of the head.

One morning, she asked me to come by before class because I was to be dispatched on a mission. I arrived at the "Adams house" an hour before class but I did not see Ida in the classroom. She was not in the kitchen either. I cautiously knocked at the door to her bedroom. She opened the door, dressed in her bathrobe, having just left the shower. Her hair was recently dried and to my surprise, it fell down her back below her waist, a fine silver mantle. I stood there, obviously at a loss. She told me to go in the kitchen and prepare some tea.

Aside from tea, the morning ritual required *The Wall Street Journal.* Ida occasionally speculated in the commodities markets and could be put into a mood that would last well into the day if *The Wall Street Journal* did not arrive on time. As she moved around a great deal, the people in the subscription department must have had a difficult time keeping track of her. As a consequence, locating a copy of *The Wall Street Journal* was a frequent activity for her assistants.

Although Ida disliked being made into a celebrity (she believed the work, not the personality, mattered), she was sometimes forced into that position in service to her desire to promote the work of "Rolfing." This often took the form of a celebration of her birthday. I remember one celebration that took place in Los Angeles. A local restaurateur had volunteered to sit on Ida's board of advisors (she was forever looking for financial advisors to help her fledgling school onto its feet). This particular year he had offered to host her birthday celebration. He operated a aspiring performers and sang or held forth in various fashions while serving the food. Poppy was his name and he had prepared a table that was a Hollywood version of a medieval feast. The table was at least twenty-five feet long and food was literally heaped on it. Waiters were singing, most at the party were ablaze with various intoxicants and, through it all, Ida sat calmly at the head of the table drinking tea. She looked as if she had walked into the scene from a Victorian movie being filmed next door. She was, however, quite at home in the chaos that surrounded her.

In 1975, Ida traveled to New York to speak at Hunter College. For the first time in public, she spoke about an "energy" that she felt was present in the body and that Rolfing helped liberate and organize. After the event, I drove her to the house of a friend, where she was to spend the night. We sat for a while talking. I mentioned that she had accomplished a great deal in her life and that I wondered what she was most proud of. Without hesitation, she said, "I am very proud of the fact that I have come up with meaningful work for people to do."

Among the many images of Ida that I carry with me, it is her hands that stand out most. Her hands were larger than most and almost simian. Years of work and arthritis had enlarged the joints and, when relaxed, her hands rested in a slight curve inward toward the palms. Sitting in class, she would work lightly on her hands with her fingernails, opening the joints and releasing the contractions of her arthritis. I see her placing her hands on a resting chest during a classroom demonstration. They lie still, almost heavy, as she comments to students. Going to work on that chest, her hands move with efficiency and strength. The power in her hands penetrates, carrying her knowledge and compassion. Those paws of hers pin the flesh and release its contractions. The chest breathes easier. Slowly she turns to the class and says, "Now it's your turn. Roll up your sleeves and get to work."

John Lodge
Ida Rolf Stories

The first time I met Ida was in my home in Boca Raton, Florida. I had learned from Bill Williams, Florida's first Rolfer, of Ida's lecture-demo to take place in Boca Raton. My wife and I invited Bill and his wife Gee Gee to bring Dr. Rolf and Rosemary Feitis to dinner at our home on the eve of the demo. It became a joyous dinner with much laughter, ghost stories, and great fun.

The demo was an extraordinary display of the Rolfing art, with hundreds in attendance seeing a young man with caved-in ribs from an auto accident stand, spread his arms and shout, "I can breathe! I can breathe!" Following that very moving moment, Dr. Rolf was surrounded by questioning people: "What do we have to do to qualify for training? How can we study with you? We want to do this work!" There were physical therapists, chiropractors, psychologists, masseurs, and laymen of all descriptions bombarding Dr. Rolf from every angle.

Bill Williams, his wife, my wife, and I stood

across the room watching. Dr. Rolf was turning back every questioner. The overview, as I remember it, was, "Your structure is not right." "You need more personal work," or something of the kind. To one very aggressive young male she said, "Go grow up!"

A husky young woman stayed and stayed, refusing refusal. "But, Dr. Rolf, I'm very strong. I've carried five-gallon milk buckets from the time I was little on the farm. And now I'm a masseuse. I work on bodies all the time." Ida looked into the person's eyes and said, "Give me your hands." After examining them, she said to the girl, "Young woman, if you want to see a Rolfer's hands, go look at that man's hands." She turned and pointed across the room to where Bill and I were standing. Of course, in my mind it was Bill she was indicating. I looked at Bill. Bill was looking at me!

I shall never forget that moment of Ida Rolf's eyes on me and that crooked finger pointing. How long we remained on that relationship, I cannot say. I was truly mesmerized. When Dr. Rolf finally turned to walk away, there were people on both sides of me holding and examining my hands! My wife was tugging at my jacket and saying, "John, do you realize what just happened?" Indeed, I did not. I was an actor and an artist. I had had no scientific background. The only thought in my head was the handshake with Ida as she left our dinner party the night before. That was the beginning.

During the three and a half years of doing drawings for the book *Rolfing,* I was reading Castaneda's books dealing with Don Juan and the shamanistic practices of Indians in Mexico. One day I said to Ida, "Wouldn't it be something to be a shaman like Don Juan?" She had read all the books. She looked at me and said. "Well, you're a shaman!" I laughed and said (thinking she was joking), "Oh, no Ida. I haven't been through the training—sorcerer's experience, tobacco juice, and fire, and all." She looked at me for some moments and in all seriousness said, "You're a shaman, because I made you one!" At which point she turned back to her writing.

One day during my practitioner training, Ida put me on the "hot spot." I was to work on a model's pelvis while she was sitting on a bench. The focus was on the sacroiliac area. It was very hot in the Adams House of Esalen where the class was being held. I was perspiring even before my trial began. With Ida's eyes focused on my work, the flood gates truly broke. It didn't go well at all. Frustrating! All at once there was a tap on my shoulder, and Ida, behind

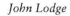

me, said, "Come on, let a good guy in there" (meaning herself). I exploded, "You're a mean old lady!" The class burst with laughter—and just as quickly stopped, sucking in their breath. The axe was about to fall! For a long moment there was dead silence. I tried to shrink into the floor. Suddenly there was ringing laughter—Ida was laughing! The class joined in. All was well. But this "shaman" has never forgotten that moment.

Years later, I was still working on drawings for the book while living and Rolfing in Santa Monica. I would fly back to New York with recent work, and Dr. Rolf would occasionally come to Los Angeles to lecture. We would get together over the latest drawings. (I had to repeat a leg drawing six times before she finally accepted it for the book. "Can't you see that it's not right? Study Dick's ankle.")

On some of her visits I would drive her to see friends that lived in the area. One lived in Orange County. When we arrived at the lady's door, we were greeted by a dachshund. The little dog had his legs splayed out behind him on the floor. He was up on his front legs with tongue out, bright eyes, and a smile on his face. But it was obvious he was in trouble. Ida asked, "What happened to doggie?" The lady responded, "Oh, Ida. Poor baby got hit by a car and I just don't have the heart to put him down." We entered and watched the brave little creature drag himself across the floor. We were seated and plied with tea and cookies. The dog stayed close to Ida, watching her. Meanwhile, the two ladies caught each other up on events and news. Suddenly Ida reached down and lifted the dog onto her lap. She stroked him and felt his pelvis as she continued talking with her friend. I was fascinated with her working hands. She returned the dog to the floor, propped him up on all four legs, and said, "Well, go ahead, try them." The dog looked bewildered as it took two steps forward with front paws, then collapsed down again in the rear. She repeated this up-and-down process three times as she continued what I have come to think of as "knitting and purling" on his spine, pelvis, and joints. She put him down finally and said, "Go on!" During her manipulation the dog had jerked his head back several times to her fingers and each time looked up at her face and smiled with his tongue out. He once again took tentative steps with his front feet— then moved a back one—then another! He was walking! He suddenly began to run! He ran circles around that living room barking at Ida each time he passed her! I had witnessed a miracle.

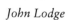

John Lodge

I don't think any of us attending that manipulation class I was in will ever forget it. There were many memorable moments, and it was the first class Peter and Emmett were jointly teaching in an adjoining space.

Upon entering promptly at 9 A.M., Ida would walk into the office, come into the class space, and wail, "Where's Rosemary?" It seemed that Rosemary followed her own timing and would appear accordingly. Meanwhile Ida, grumbling, would begin the class. One morning a student made a remark about Rosemary's lateness. Ida stopped, faced the class, and said, "Rosemary can do more in half an hour than you could do in four hours!"

That was Ida!

June Schwartz

When I first started thinking about Ida for this effort, I was drawn to certain notions about her that have to do with the importance of her work, her rigor, her magic vision often without seeming to look, and her scorn when we didn't live up to her idea of what we should be doing.

Now my recurrent images are softer, usually of her womanliness, a hand straying up to tuck a loose strand into her hairdo, patting a flower in her hair or fingering a brooch at her neckline, her pleasure at the prospect of a good meal.

I was having a session with Ida in her New York apartment and asked what she thought of my daughter starting sessions with Hadidjah Lamas. She looked at Lisa for a moment, then fixed her attention on Dana, my younger daughter, and announced, "*She's* the one who needs work." Dana remembers her fear of this crone's fierce eyes, and of Ida's crooked finger pointing at her; she was afraid of the sessions.

Ida turned back to Lisa and asserted, "*You* should do something in life with your hands," and poked about in a bookcase for a copy of *Hands* for Lisa to look at.

A few years later, Dana was a model in the advanced class Ida was teaching in Joe Adams' house in Big Sur. Dana was seated on a bench, with Beverly Silverman's hands working on one side, and Al Drucker on the other. Ida's gaze was to the outside, and without turning her head, she instructed Beverly and Al precisely where their hands should be to effect the change she wanted.

Thanks for this opportunity to reflect and write about Ida. All the years I've thought about her, I've focused on her work, her effect on me and my family, our work together in the Education Committee, and always her tough side was uppermost for me. Not until this past few weeks did I give proper place in my own memory to the womanly, tender side of the great Ida P. Rolf.

Gene Man

I remember being Rolfed by Ida. "When did you have your accident?" she said. "I didn't have an accident," said I. "You must have," she replied. "God didn't give you that rib cage." Next day, suddenly the conversation came back to me and I said to myself, of course I had an accident. I was about ten years old when I got hit by a bobsled. It knocked the wind out of me and made me a little sore, but I forgot about it until Ida's very knowledgeable fingers found it.

Another memory: I brought together a distinguished group of scientists, really an impeccable group, who were also open-minded about Rolfing and non-traditional healing. They were going to help with research into Rolfing; all agreed to go through Rolfing, that was part of the deal. To start, they would be introduced to the process by a lecture-demonstration. One of them was a biophysicist, I believe from Baylor

University, who weighed about 250 pounds. In the demonstration portion of the program, Ida assigned him to her son, who weighed about the same, for Rolfing. The rest of the team watched an interaction and output of energy between Rolfer and Rolfee second only to the WWII atom bomb as, with cursing and sweating, they heaved their way through a first session. Nevertheless, the group did all complete their Rolfing.

Valerie V. Hunt, ED.D.
Reminiscences of Ida Rolf

One day in the late 1960s some of my physiology students, who were also dancers, asked me to explain what was occurring in Rolfing. From their description of what happened during their Rolfing sessions, I couldn't explain it. Excitedly they told me that their dancing had improved, they were more relaxed, and they had altered states of consciousness. Some days later, I recorded one of the dancers using telemetry, electromyography, EMG. The recordings showed strange happenings in their muscles that were not explained by physiology.

A few days later, I attended a meeting at the University sponsored by the dance department where Ida Rolf gave a lecture. At that time I directed the Division of Physical Therapy and was well acquainted with manipulative techniques, although not with Rolfing. I listened to Ida and saw her demonstration but still couldn't understand what happened. After the lecture I spoke with Ida, telling her about my EMG findings. She excitedly asked what those

Valerie V. Hunt, ED.D

recordings meant. When I told her I didn't know, she answered with, "Well, find out! You find out and I will find the money to sponsor your research," straight and to the point as Ida always was. Two years later I produced a project report: "A Study of Structural Integration from Neuromuscular, Energy Field, and Emotional Approaches." Reprints of this report are still available at the Rolf Institute. For me this report completely changed the direction of my research to study Human Energy Fields.

Twenty-five years later my findings are reported in my new book *Infinite Mind: The Science of Human Vibrations*. The research that was born the day that Ida commanded that I "go find out" has contributed important information to all hands-on therapy, sound and light treatments, and alternative medicine.

Thanks, Ida Rolf, for your insight and convictions and for your impelling strength that altered my life's work.

Gaining Momentum

(1970 – 1973)

Karl E. Humiston
Memories of Ida Rolf

Only once did I experience Ida's hands personally Rolfing me, and that was for less than a minute. During my auditing, in May-June 1971 in Big Sur, California, I received four post-ten sessions from a practitioner trainee, under her watchful eye and direction. Most of the work was on my feet, and all of it was for me a very intense experience, usually leaving me drenched and so exhausted that I would leave the class to sleep an hour or so. Once, while watching my session, she said, "Here, let me show you," and slowly lumbered from her chair to the stool at my feet. She applied her knuckle to my sole, a stick of dynamite exploded inside my foot, and she lumbered back to her seat. For me, no one else's Rolfing touch has ever come near to hers.

During that same training, I remained in the classroom during a lunch break while she interviewed a young man who was requesting admission to training. After a few minutes of talk, she said she would not accept him into Rolf training, adding, "You are an angry young man, and I will not allow angry people to do my work on other people's bodies." Obviously irritated, he demanded to know why she thought he was an angry person. She said simply, "I can see."

At least once during the training, after she made one of her profound observations about the subject being worked on, someone asked, "Ida, how do you know that?" With a trace of frustration in her voice, she answered, "Well, look!"

Michael Baker

An Account of Events Leading Up To and Including My First Encounter With Ida Rolf

"What's that?" I said, in response to the strange statement: "I've just been Rolfed," coming from the young man across the dining room table. "It's something invented by Ida Rolf; it lines you up and clears out obsolete muscular patterns. I've just had my first session and for the first time in years, I feel like I am breathing." Just before this strange interruption, I had been quietly sitting in the dining room of Esalen, holding a warm mug of tea and staring out the window at the garden and the ocean, during an afternoon break from a workshop on Gestalt Therapy run by Fritz Perls. As I was the only one in the dining room at the time, I was the chosen outlet for the explosion of feelings that needed to be expressed by this young man—who at the time was a medical student at UC San Francisco—after his first Rolfing session, a transforming experience for him. And it would transform me and my life, although I did not know it at the time, nor appreciate my luck at being "chosen," even as I listened to his description of how his sternum opened up, his thorax opened up, and, most important, how he opened up. Like many of us after the first revelatory Rolfing session, he babbled on and on with a vitality and excitement that was infectious and inspiring.

After the weekend, I returned to Stanford, where I was doing postdoctoral studies on nerve growth factor protein in the Genetics Department, and thought about getting Rolfed. It was 1970. The energy and ferment of the late 1960s and early 1970s were in full flower on the Stanford Campus, including demonstrations against the Vietnam War. At the time, many creative (and not so creative) New Age therapies were being born and spread throughout the Bay Area. And at the same time, I was making a transition from engineering to biology, while struggling to keep a four-year-old marriage together.

With my analytical mindset, a result of a number of years of education in engineering, bodywork as a path for personal growth or even as important for general well-being seemed foreign to me. My mind and intellect seemed to be a more fertile focus for learning and for achieving a fuller and more satisfying life. I remember talking about Rolfing with an M.D. in our lab who told me that Rolfing wouldn't harm me but also it wouldn't help. And so I put the idea into the background as I struggled with my everyday problems and tasks.

Of course, all this meant was that the idea of getting Rolfed needed time to germinate and grow inside of me, as I matured and explored other forms of personal growth available in the Bay Area. It took a crisis in my life a year later, when it seemed like my center could not hold together, to motivate me to get Rolfed. And as I went through the Rolfing process, I discovered my center in the deepest and most meaningful way.

At the time, I did not even remotely dream of becoming a Rolfer. However, being Rolfed stimulated me to take body movement and dance workshops, learn massage and, most important, to appreciate how my body's structure and responses to the world are central to all aspects of my life. Even my science became more creative and productive.

About a year later, I learned about a weekend workshop by Ida Rolf in Berkeley; I think it was in a lecture hall at a theological school. The workshop consisted of a demonstration of two Rolfing sessions and an opportunity to experience exercises designed for people who had been Rolfed. Out of curiosity about the exercises and also to see Ida Rolf in action, but without any other strong intention, I signed up and went up to Berkeley. The first morning began with Emmett Hutchins doing a first hour on a model under Ida's supervision. It made Rolfing seem even more mysterious. At the same time, I began to appreciate more how wonderful and powerful was Ida's gift to us.

When we returned after lunch, Ida told everyone to get into their underwear, a surprise to me and I think to most of the participants, many of whom were therapists who were not comfortable with their bodies. But Ida said, and we did; no questions were allowed, no dissent was even considered. So there we were, on our backs in our underwear, moving our elbows in and out, or our feet towards our heads, or rolling our heads from side to side, etc. What an unexpected development! The next day, Emmett did a second hour on the model. I began to see a small part of the postural changes in the model and became even more excited about Rolfing. And I began to wish that I could learn this skill. At one of the breaks, I went near Ida to listen to questions she received and heard many requests to be trained as a Rolfer. She would look at each person, examine their hands, ask a few questions, and usually (almost always) say no. Pleading with Ida did not work. It was a steady line of applicants, with most being rejected.

Nevertheless, my desire to learn to give others something of what I received from Rolfing was so strong that at the end of the workshops I screwed up my courage and went over to her. I told her I was interested in becoming a Rolfer. Without any look of encouragement, she asked me why and also lifted up my hands to examine them. As I sputtered out a response of how important Rolfing was to me and how much I wanted to give this experience to others, she dropped my hands and had a look that appeared to me to be one of disgust, as if my hands were incapable of holding a glass of water, let alone doing the hard work of Rolfing. She asked about my background, and I told her about my biochemistry research. With a sigh of a suffering teacher, who is martyred by having to put up with mediocre material to train, she turned to her assistant and said something like, "He'll do."

So, Ida Rolf, trained at the early part of the twentieth century in biochemistry, was inviting me to learn her process for helping people to rediscover their body and reclaim this heritage as an essential part of living. I, an engineer turned biochemist, was to become a Rolfer and begin a journey that would lead me along a path of discovery and understanding that would be the transforming experience of my life.

Don Hanlon Johnson
Two Memories

After auditing with Ida at Esalen the summer of 1971, I did my first training class with her at the University of Florida's Pigeon Key during that fall. Her assistant was her son, Dick Demmerle, the first time he had participated in her new format for teaching people outside the community of osteopaths. I had a series of dreams either about Ida herself or about my own Rolfing sessions, which I told to Ida every day to her delight. She often used them as clues in working with me. I had such a dream on the eve of Thanksgiving, which all of us were celebrating together on this swampy, four-acre man-made plot situated directly underneath the causeway to Key West. We began preparing for the dinner in the late afternoon. Rosemary, as I recall, was the chief cook. John Lodge, Doug Wallace (God rest his beautiful soul!), and I began drinking wine and taking other substances. By the time the turkey was done, much later than we had anticipated, the three of us had drifted into something of a rap group, whose subjects were our class, its foibles, and particular quirks in its life together. Ida's obvious enjoyment of our ensemble spurred us forward to the dangerous edge where I was sober enough to stop for just a moment to ask myself, should I really tell this latest dream? I dared to proceed: In my dream I saw a vast barren battlefield in a strange country named "Rolfing." Two armies were amassed face-to-face like in old Hollywood movies. One army was led by Ida with John Lodge as her general; the other, by Dick Demmerle. They were about to engage in battle to decide who would reign over the country. I awoke not knowing who won. There was a ghastly silence, furtive glances here and there. I was sure I had tripped over the edge into forbidden territory. Suddenly Ida burst into raucous laughter and we all joined her in relief. The party went on.

During Ida's final years, I sat on the Board of Directors. The last time I saw her was at a meeting in New York at the office on 91st Street, during which we finalized our negotiations for the Institute's right to use and inherit her name in its service marks. It was a hard day for her. By then, she was confined to a wheelchair and not feeling well. Here she had to confront giving up rights connected with her very identity and the family issues related to it. We adjourned late in the afternoon agreeing to meet later for dinner at a seafood restaurant a block or so away on

Amsterdam. For some reason, it turned out that I was left alone with her while others went elsewhere before coming back for dinner. She asked me to wheel her the short distance to the restaurant. We were quiet together. We got a table; it was early enough so the restaurant was virtually empty. There was a shellfish bar. The rest of our group would not show up for an hour. Ida ordered mussels. Because I grew up in California where mussels were quarantined for most of my youth, I had never eaten any; this was the first time. When I told her that, she began telling me stories of when she was a little girl on Long Island and would go with her father early in the morning to gather mussels. We wove together stories of our childhood years. We sat together in silence. I felt deep affection for her. This was the last time I saw her.

Joseph Heller

During my practitioner training, my partner was digging in my rib cage on a third session when Ida came out with one of her statements: "You are not going to get it there!" I felt Roger tense as he realized this was addressed to him. He fumbled for a few minutes and then Ida stood up and regally came over to my table. I was lying on my side with my back to her, but I felt her approaching. Suddenly her elbow landed on the side of my ribs and I went berserk. Every part of my body was flailing except for the part under her elbow. Then, as abruptly as it started, it stopped. In relief I took a breath so deep that I could hardly believe it. Apparently it was visible to the class that had by then assembled around my table, because several of them gasped and someone said, "Jesus!" to which Ida smilingly replied, "No! Ida!"

I was driving Dr. Rolf to the Los Angeles airport for

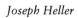

Joseph Heller

her return home. At that time Ida was walking on her own with a cane, so you can imagine my surprise when we pulled up to the curb and Ida said, "Get me a wheelchair and a black porter." I had by then learned not to argue, so I came back with a wheelchair, which she promptly occupied, and a black porter who took her bags and ushered us through the various stations. When we got to the gate the attendants said to be ready because they would be loading her first. As we stood waiting, Ida turned to me and said, "I learned a long time ago that the way to get through an airport is with a black porter and a wheelchair."

We were at a gathering of Rolfers and I watched Dr. Rolf respond to several Rolfers who were inquiring about becoming teachers with an emphatic "Never!" After we were alone, I asked her how come she did that when some of them looked like potential candidates. She said, "Listen! If all it takes to discourage them is one word from me, they don't deserve to be teachers."

Owen James
Ida Rolf's Red Geranium

It was just our luck that there were geraniums around our house. You know Ida had to have one for her hair each day. She took the time to fix her hair into its up position and then garnish it with red, and be on time for the nine o'clock start that I wasn't always there for. Somehow it always took me a little extra time to get there from Barbara's little house with the Buddha meditating in view of Burns' Creek bridge. I found this a particularly painful class, so caring for the geraniums was a great relief. Ida must have caught on, as she suggested one day that maybe I should become a gardener instead of a Rolfer. She did have a way of hitting the mark.

After watching all that squirming around on the tables during class I just had to get outside. After all, down the road were all the encounter screamers and Fritz helping people to get it out. There was Murano's class acting out all the roles, and that got pretty noisy sometimes. There was Bernie Gunther jumping with joy out on the lawn. A couple of

Owen James

psychiatrists in that Rolfing class never did practice Rolfing. Fritz sent a few over to get them into their bodies but I think they got scared out of their skin. It was popular in those early days to make a lot of noise while being Rolfed.

This reminds me of one of my very first weeks working at the baths at Esalen. I'm three weeks out of class and yet another first hour to do. For three weeks I have done only first hours and a couple of second hours. This fellow, as soon as my hand touches his skin, screams out. Soon after that I was given a room on the second tier, far from the Esalen dining room.

My fondest memories of Ida were the quick glances I would take of her as she sipped her morning coffee or paused between sentences during her class lectures. I was in awe of her. Even the way she held her head in thought touched me. She was gracious at one moment and searingly truthful at another. Often the long afternoons of writhing models and perspiring practitioners were interrupted with her fiery statement of "No! No! No! NOT THERE! HERE!" She could blister a student with a comment about their work and then on her way out she would touch them on the shoulder and one knew it was all right . . . for the moment.

Undoubtedly one of her persistent problems was getting us to understand what she was conveying to us. "Six hundred and one times!"—she would bellow in mock exhaustion. "I tell you students something at least six hundred times and the six hundred and first time now you tell me as if you just discovered it." One learned how to listen in her classes.

I was a bit disheartened as her eyesight failed

when she began to call me Ed Taylor, and yet I suspected she was seeing only the contour of the individual. I reasoned that Ed and I looked a lot alike. And we did. We are almost the same height, have reddish curly hair, and similar shoulder girdles. I would have felt better if she called Ed Taylor Neal Powers, but alas she called Ed Taylor Ed Taylor and me Ed Taylor. I figured it was another gift of humility.

I remember attending her funeral in Philadelphia and looking down at those magnificent hands that sculpted so many people. They were the hands of a woman, an artist, and a worker.

As an early student of hers I was never quite certain how to work, yet in her presence I felt I could do no harm. She gifted many of us with individual insights that continue to guide our work over the years. "Top of the head up, waistline back" she would insist. And "Roll up your sleeves and get to work." Many of her comments became ingrained in us as new and healthy habit patterns. I am forever grateful to her. Her lectures on Rolfing lit a fire of inquiry that continues to inspire me. When I first encountered Ida and her work, I knew immediately it was my life's work. I continue on this path with the deepest respect and love for Dr. Rolf. I am also deeply appreciative of the wonderful times I share with my colleagues.

— *Neal Powers a.k.a. Ed Taylor*

Tom West

Since I went through basic and advanced training with Ida in 1973 and 1974, I had many "encounters" with her. I saw her with the extremes of emotion— very happy when her advanced class threw a surprise birthday party for her (sitting in a chair with a rose in her hair and a glass of wine at her side opening presents with all her loving and caring students sitting on the floor looking up at her). And her deep sadness when her favorite Rolfer in Florida was caught in a serious indiscretion and left the Institute.

I remember she once got mad at me for being two days late for her advanced training class. I had to stay in Florida for graduation at my college. For three days she would not acknowledge I had arrived and was in the class. I got mad back and would not even look at her. Finally she looked at me and said, "I see Tom has decided to be with us. Tom, what can you tell us about the vertical line?" My answer didn't please her but the thaw happened.

Much later in the class, she invited me to her

home for dinner. I was thrilled to death, since I idolized her, but it turned out to be very uncomfortable since I didn't know how to carry on a conversation with her other than Rolfing. I had identified her so strongly with it that I couldn't imagine what else we could talk about—especially when I remembered the time she first met me and I proudly announced I was a psychologist. She looked at me with annoyance and said, "There's no such thing as psychology—it's all in the body!"

One of the most frightening times was when we had a very outspoken Rolf candidate visit my practitioner class. He asked if the Rolfing process produced tangible and observable changes with each session. Ida firmly said certainly and anyone in the practitioner class could easily judge what session a Rolfee had completed by looking at her/him. The candidate asked for proof with a demonstration while all of us were shaking in our boots—especially when Ida stated that if we couldn't judge the hour we shouldn't be in the class. The sigh of relief was very obvious when she decided not to let him have his demonstration. Needless to say, he was not accepted for training.

When she observed you working on someone during training and you would turn to her and ask how you were doing, the best you could get from her was, "It's better." That would make you feel like you had hung the moon! I did consider her like a mother or grandmother to me. This brought out my rebellion, deep dependency, love/hate, worship, and tremendous respect. To meet her and decide to move into Rolfing—even though I had a full professional career going—was one of the very best decisions I have ever made. She is still a wonderful part of my life. She will always live on!

Charles Siemers
Pelvic Lift Story

Some time ago, there was spirited discussion in *Rolf Lines* on the pelvic lift. The following IPR story may well add to general understanding of the pelvic lift. Well, when IPR gave a pelvic lift, the client's pelvis was a foot off the table and she rocked it powerfully. It was like trying to hang on to a bucking bronco. Those psoas were activated like pistons pumping energy through the whole being. Some old-time Rolfers believe that Rolfing was born out of IPR finding and mastering the psoas!

I was sitting in practitioners class next to IPR. Late in the afternoon she looked out through a window at the mountains and brought the freshness and vitality of the nature into her. I shared her experience simply by sitting next to her.

Seeing Story

One afternoon I was assisting IPR in an advanced class. I began experiencing an awareness of the Rolfing sessions. My head would just turn automatically to one of the Rolfing sessions being done and I would just see what was needed in that moment. I mentioned this enlightening experience to IPR and she said, "That's the way I do it, don't tell anyone!"

I remember while I was assisting IPR in an advanced class, one of my jobs was at three o'clock every day. I was to prepare and bring IPR's coffee. It was made with cream and made exactly the same every day. Well, on the way over on the first day, I hear and feel this growl coming at me on the inner planes. Something about my right hip didn't seem to exactly please her!

That night, and every night for the next few weeks, I began poking around on myself on Peter Melchior's living room floor—and every day at three o'clock, with coffee in hand, I felt that same growl coming from IPR about some imbalance in me.

During those first few weeks, there was a lot of talk among the students about energy, but I didn't hear a word about it from IPR. Finally one day I'm on the ritual coffee delivery and I feel this great internal smile and warmth filling me.

The next morning in class, IPR points at me. "Look at Chuck. He looks pretty integrated and nobody's laid a hand on him; must be that integrating energy in the room." From there, she launched into a commanding discussion on elbows and integration, a discourse that left us with enough "food for thought" to last a lifetime.

I can tell you, as we all knew, she had perceptions and communication beyond the ordinary. Over two decades later, I can still feel the energy of her growl, and the warmth of her smile.

Jim Lewis

One Friday after class, we had an informal dance social planned. Folks wandered in, had a drink, chatted, started dancing. Dr. Rolf arrived; she sat herself in a corner and started expounding on her philosophy. A couple of us began to listen, then a few more; finally, most of us were in the corner listening. So much for the party! She never lost an opportunity to expand our appreciation and understanding of the work.

In the advanced class of 1974, we were reviewing the third hour. I was working around the crest of the ilium and having a little trouble getting in. Dr. Rolf came over and said, "Step aside." She put her fingers in and worked for a minute or two. Then she said, "That's what you're looking for." I put my fingers back on the body, and it was as if I had fallen into a hole. There was clarity and differentiation. I'll never forget that experience.

Also during the '74 advanced class, one Rolfer had a delusional episode. He put Dr. Rolf's sweater over his shoulders, sat in her chair, and began to direct the Rolfing class as if he were her. She stayed on the sidelines and let him proceed, saying that he was totally accurate in his perceptions. Later in the day, the situation got a bit more bizarre with paranoia about safety—ours and Dr. Rolf's—setting in.

I remember being worked on by a classmate—I believe Don Johnson—upstairs in a hallway, with Dr. Rolf giving suggestions on the fly. It was really stressful to have received the session under those circumstances, and afterwards I asked Dr. Rolf for help as I didn't feel well with the work. She laid me on my side and put her elbow into my ribs and axilla. I asked what she was doing and she said that this is what she always did to rebalance the shoulder girdle. It felt great!

I also remember one model Dr. Rolf worked on. She had cerebral palsy and hadn't been on her feet without human support for over ten years. The foot work was extremely painful but the client was determined. At the last session, she arrived by taxi and with the aid of hand walkers she walked up the path and into the classroom. It was a very moving moment.

Louis Schultz
Reflections on Ida Rolf

First of all, I will say that I never called Dr. Rolf "Ida" to her face. When I grew up you didn't call an elder by their first name unless they asked you to— and she never did.

I first met Dr. Rolf at a selection meeting in Boulder in 1972. In those days the selection was on Saturday and next Monday you were either in the class or looking for something else to do for the next six weeks. Richard Stenstadvold had suggested that I come up to meet her since I was having thoughts about applying to become a Rolfer. She told me that I should never do bioenergetics and Rolfing at the same time (which I was doing) and asked if I were interested in teaching anatomy for the Guild (which is what the organization was called at that time). I later found out that was my selection!

About six months after I trained, I suggested the idea of a week of anatomy review before the Rolfing training. Dr. Rolf was emphatic that I could not do this without doing the advanced training. Since it was much too soon after my basic training, she allowed me to audit the advanced. In those days, the advanced training was six weeks reviewing the basic ten sessions and then a month of advanced work. During the last part, fascial anatomy was presented. The Rolfer who normally gave this part couldn't do it so the day before the advanced part of the class she informed me that I was presenting the material on fascia. There was a frantic development of the body stocking idea, which seemed to please everyone and was a relief to me. Later I traveled to different regions to present these concepts to Rolfers who hadn't had it. I can remember driving across the western United States from Denver to California listening to the tapes of my lectures. I didn't want to hear me (I hate listening to myself), but I wanted her comments, which were always pertinent and different from the way I had been thinking.

During that advanced training in 1974, the Rolfers were, of course, always looking for Dr. Rolf's approval (rarely given, if at all). One Rolfer was working with a young man who was extremely squeamish and complaining. The Rolfer was trying to work on the ankle maleoli and Dr. Rolf kept saying that the Rolfer was not getting it done. The harder the Rolfer worked, the more the young man squirmed. Finally in exasperation, Dr. Rolf got out of her chair (I think it was before the wheelchair), sort of lurched over to the table, and came down with a knuckle on either maleolus. The man gasped wordlessly. Dr. Rolf looked down at him and said, "I think that will change your opinion of little old ladies."

In that same advanced training, Dr. Rolf did a demonstration on a woman with cerebral palsy who had never walked. At one point Dr. Rolf was kneeling on the bed going down the woman's back. The woman slid off the bed. Dr. Rolf then peered over the edge of the table and said, "Now Marjory, see if you can bring your waistline back."

In early 1976, Ron Thompson, Jim Asher, and I did a dissection in Philadelphia. After a number of weeks, we felt that we had demonstrated enough to invite Dr. Rolf to view our splendid work and to look at Ron's magnificent slides. She was wheeled in by Dick Demmerle and could see the top of the head of our cadaver (the head had not yet been dissected). From the swirls of hair and other observations, she described the entire body including rotations and other variations. Humbly we took the rest of the afternoon off. . . .

When I did my advanced training in New Jersey en route to my move to New York City, I decided to start using my middle name. When I told Dr. Rolf, she said, "Good! I've got enough Dicks in my life."

From that day on she was the only one in the class who never missed on using my name.

In my advanced training in 1976, there were ten males in the class. Very few if any of us wore underwear. Each time that Dr. Rolf called for a lineup, there would be a mad scramble in the corner with briefs coming out of brief cases, lunch bags, coat pockets, backpacks, or off a shelf. Dr. Rolf, of course, had no patience and would yell, "I told you that you were to be ready to line up at all times." After a while, we wore her down and she sat grumpily while we prepared ourselves for public examination.

A related story I have heard happened in a class at Esalen. When Dr. Rolf called for a class lineup, everyone did—naked. She took one look and yelled, "Put on your underwear!"

Dr. Rolf and I had very little social interaction. One time for some reason, she came to my apartment for dinner. Because she said she liked it, I made corned beef and cabbage (something I had never made before). She praised the meal. She said, "You cut the corned beef in big chunks which I like—those girls always slice it so thin." Of course it was big chunks because I didn't know any better. I later fed her the same meal again—never change success—and she was just as happy.

Once when I was being a model in an advanced

class, the Rolfer was trying to work on the inside of my rami. Dr. Rolf kept saying "deeper, deeper" and I was saying "deeper" (to get it over with). My Rolfer was sweating, saying, "I've never been this deep in the perineum." Finally, in exasperation, Dr. Rolf came over and did indeed go deeper inside my rami. She then looked at my Rolfer and said, "Can you do the other side or must I do that also?" With much effort, mumbling, and sweating, the other side was accomplished. This may be why this area has been such a focus for me ever since.

In another class, Dr. Rolf was helping a student Rolfer work on the groin region of a very well endowed young man. This quite covered the area she wanted to work in and we all wondered what she would do. She looked for a while and finally said, "Would you move your movables?" He did and the work went on.

Dr. Rolf did not do much work on me. Occasionally when I was suffering lower back pain, she would sit me down and do what I called her "chicken scratches" on my lower back and say, "There," and I was better. Once she was helping a Rolfer work behind my ear. This seemed to go on forever. After she finished, the students asked in awe, "How did that feel?" My comment, still hurting, was, "She has the longest damn fingernails I've ever felt."

Whenever I was in the neighborhood of one of Dr. Rolf's classes, she assumed that I would be available to give a lecture. It was not, "Will you . . ." but rather, "You will. . . ." One time I was traveling to do some Rolfing in Los Angeles with a very full schedule. Dr. Rolf was teaching there and Jim Asher was assisting her. I arranged to have a session with Jim after the class. I arrived late, hoping to miss seeing Dr. Rolf, but she was still there. Upon seeing me she said something like, "Good! You can give a lecture tomorrow morning in the class." I told her, "No, I have too much work to do with clients." It was in a motel room where the kitchen was divided from the main room by a high counter. She stood on one side of the counter firmly nodding "Yes" while I, on the other side, was shaking my head "No." This went on in silence and the entire class was silent, watching. When she saw that this was not going to work, she lapsed into a little old lady routine, saying, "Nobody tells me anything—I didn't know that you were going to be here." I did not give the lecture. . . .

When I first got to know Dr. Rolf, she wanted me to do a hundred things for her, none of which would have provided an income. I finally said, "What is the one thing you want me to do?" She said, "Write a book on fascial anatomy." When I couldn't get started for a couple of years, she finally said, "Write the book with Rosemary." Some twenty years later we have completed the book and I can finally not feel Dr. Rolf hovering over my shoulder with that *look* she always had when you were not doing things her way. I am deeply indebted to her for a whole new direction to my life.

Rolf Institute
(1974 to present)

Richard Stenstadvold

Dr. Rolf's "No Nonsense" Way
of Looking at Life

One snowy day in Boulder, I was taking Dr. Rolf to the Denver airport so she could fly home to the East Coast. Because the weather was quite bad, I drove her in our Toyota Land Cruiser.

I had never told Dr. Rolf of my serious problem with directions and how easily I could get lost. I have absolutely no sense of North, South, East, or West. Accordingly, I have to memorize how to get from one place to another.

When I got to the airport exit on the freeway, a large truck had overturned in the snowstorm. The exit was closed. I panicked, since I didn't know how to get to the airport other than using the blocked exit. As I drove past the airport exit, I explained to Dr. Rolf the serious problem I had with directions. Her response? She told me, "Take the next exit . . . pull over . . . stand on top of the jeep to see which way the airplanes are landing . . . and head off in that direction." That's what I did, and sure enough, together, we found the airport.

Dean Rollings

In 1969 I moved to Esalen Institute in Big Sur, California, to study Gestalt Therapy with Fritz Perls. This was an exciting time—the birth of contemporary psychology had begun with such notables as John Lilly, Alan Watts, Jack Downing, Dick Price, Will Schultz, Oscar Ichazo, Gregory Bateson, and others who experimented in the evolution of therapy beyond Freud. It was Fritz Perls who was responsible for bringing Ida Rolf to Esalen.

One of the most visible and interesting developments of that time at Esalen was the work of Dr. Rolf. Her theory that physical structure has a role in evolution and mental health influenced the work of practically everyone at Esalen. Exciting research was begun at Agnew State Hospital on the effect of Rolfing. This study was designed by Julian Silverman, Ida Rolf, and Valerie Hunt. Reports of the fascinating effects of her work spread rapidly throughout the field of psychiatry.

It was Ida's statement "There is no psychology,

only the body," that changed the course of my life. Peter and Emmett had just moved to Boulder, so I returned to Colorado where I trained as a Rolfer and practiced until the next time Ida and I met. In 1976 I was accepted into Ida's advanced class in New Jersey with her son Dick Demmerle. Upon arriving for the first day of class with a full-blown case of Rocky Mountain tick fever and not having slept for what seemed like days, I was asked by Ida to do a demonstration for a group of press people. This was to be one of the most humbling experiences of my life. A short while into the session Ida asked me to explain the pattern in the chest and its probable cause. I responded in true Esalen style by asking whether she wanted a physical or emotional explanation. "Just explain it!" she snapped. OK, now it was time to take me apart and well she did. Ida would not hear of my talking of emotional patterns and the type of life experience that could account for this structure. Now she began to criticize and correct every move I made. She suddenly stopped me with the model totally unbalanced and ended the session. I was in disbelief at her behavior and confronted her to no avail. End of Day One. On Day Two, and for the next two and a half months, I generally did the first demonstration model. Once Ida made me do a model working on the carpeted floor until my knuckles bled. It was trial by fire! No one had ever treated me the way Ida Rolf did, and there were a number of strong and angry confrontations between us. One of these conflicts became so intense that several Rolfers took it upon themselves to get between Ida and me and break us up.

Ida's teaching was as much about semantics as it was about Rolfing. In the last week of class she invited me over for tea. It was then that she told me it was not the words she had spoken but the emotions and spaces she had put me through that I had needed to learn. I understood that she was absolutely right! From that point to the end of her life, we would be close friends.

After the class, I returned to Boulder where Joseph Heller (who had just been appointed President of the Rolf Institute by Ida) came over to meet me. Soon I was appointed Vice President and we were off to bring Rolfing into the world. One of our first projects was to set up speaking engagements for Ida throughout the country. These began to draw a large number of people and her ideas and fame spread. At the same time, research remained a priority for Ida. The project she had in mind was to take a community of people, do a base study on them, and then have them Rolfed to see if integrated structure would translate into social change. To find financial support for this study, I approached my uncle James Ivy, who at that time was Executive Vice President of the Ford Foundation. We subsequently had several meetings. After the first presentation, Ida suddenly approached my uncle, threw him down on the sofa, and commenced to Rolf him for the duration of the afternoon. Ida's proposal was given serious consideration by the Board of Directors of the Foundation. In the end they decided, unfortunately, that it failed to fit into the type of projects they were chartered to fund.

Ida's health was beginning to fail and she wished to teach what was to be one of her last classes. The class was called Advance Two and was held at Brugh Joy's Ranch in the Mojave Desert. I had the good fortune to be one of the twelve people invited. We were to spend the next six weeks in isolation. It was one of the richest periods I have spent in my life. There were too many experiences to write of now but I want to mention a few highlights:

Ida's birthday, when all she wanted to do was Rolf children and children she Rolfed—what may have been the whole child population of the Mojave Desert.

Seeing her pleasure at receiving the first copy of her book—years in the making.

Working with acoustic and electromagnetic fields with Rolfing.

Analyzing the data of UCLA research with Val
Hunt and Roslyn Bruyere.

Long and very fast drives through the desert with
Ida in my 300 SL 6.3 which, by the way, was one of
Ida's favorite diversions in life. She said that she used
to take drives to contemplate and meditate. She very
much missed being able to drive herself in later life.

Flying Ida in a helicopter to ancient Indian ruins
and hot springs.

And so it was—a great time with a grand lady.

After leaving the ranch we went to San Francisco
where Ida's eightieth birthday was to be celebrated
at the St. Francis Yacht Club. Hundreds of people
with lighted candles in hand met her, wishing her a
happy birthday. Ida Rolf was now being seen as a
great teacher. She would not indulge in the opportunity to be idolized. One of her favorite sayings in
these situations was, "Roll up your sleeves and let's
get to work."

The following spring Marshal Thurber began the
first Burklin School for Business, which was billed as
a New Age school and the first of its kind, in Ver-
mont. The school had many instructors who came
from all over the world. Among the notables was
Bucky Fuller. He and Ida speculated on the tensegrity
model of the human structure. Some years earlier,
when Bucky was with Ida at some get-together, he

made the claim that he would show her how to change structure. He assumed a military pose and said, "That's how you change structure." It was during Burklin that he apologized for this statement. By the way, Bucky came to see Ida shortly before her death to pay his respects.

During Ida's stay at Burklin, Marshal Thurber and Joe Heller proposed to her that they buy the rights to Rolfing for one million dollars. This was a time of turmoil for Rolfing. The Rolf Institute wanted to acquire the rights to the name and the body of knowledge. Dr. Rolf was affronted by some members of the Institute who felt that she had no right to appoint Joe Heller as President. Chaos ran wild and there was the possibility that there would be no Rolfing organization to carry on her work. It was very disturbing. It was during one of those heated times, I remember, that Ida said to me, "I wonder if Rolfing works, if this type of behavior is coming from the supposed best examples, the practitioners." I said to her, "It's hard to form an organization when you are so good at making individuals." She had to laugh.

The offer to buy the rights to Rolfing weighed heavily on Ida. She knew that time was growing short. I spent many hours discussing this with Ida as did Joe and Marshal. I had a number of strong interactions with both of them. In the end, Ida decided that the work belonged to the people she had taught, the Rolf Institute.

I returned to New York not long after Ida Rolf went into a convalescent home in New Jersey. I visited with her every few weeks until her death. I know she left this earth with a feeling of completion and satisfaction.

Jason Mixter
Letter to My Children

Dearest Children,

Two of you have just turned six years old, my dear twins Camille and Meredith; and Willie, you have just turned two. I have no idea when you will read this or whether you will be able to extract any meaning from it, but I do want you to know about someone who was (and still is) very important to Daddy. I hope that by reading this you may one day understand that life-transforming people can and often do enter your lives when you least expect it, for this is exactly what happened to me at a time in my life when things looked pretty bleak. Her name was Ida Pauline Rolf and I will never forget her.

In 1971, I found myself at a place called the Esalen Institute, which hangs high on a cliff above the Pacific Ocean in Big Sur, California. I was freshly graduated from college, had hardly traveled west of Worcester, Massachusetts, and on one level, thought I was pretty cool; yet on another level, I was confused, lost, and fearful that I would never find my path, my life's work. At twenty-four I had already failed at my childhood dream of becoming a neurosurgeon. Looking back, I guess I wasn't cut out to spend long hours peering through a microscope in some dimly lit laboratory, conducting experiments in which I was supposed to achieve the exact same results that countless others had achieved before me. Back then I concluded that not pursuing a medical career was proof that I would never measure up to my family's or anyone's expectations and proved that I was fundamentally defective.

After changing my major from premed to government, I ran a very successful business for the rest of my undergraduate years. Junior year, I accepted an offer from Alcoa Aluminum to pay my way through Harvard Business School if I agreed to work for them a minimum of two years after graduate school. It wasn't neurosurgery but I thought it would have to do.

Around that time, the 1960s hit your daddy full in the face. I marched against the Vietnam war, practiced yoga and meditation, grew my hair down my back, and subsequently backed out of the deal with Alcoa. I packed up my VW bus and headed for California. I was going to Esalen Institute, which promised emotional breakthroughs through Gestalt and Encounter group therapy, sexual freedom, communal nudity, yoga and meditation instruction, and intense body therapies like Rolfing and Neo-Reichian work. I hoped to find a convincing alternative to the gospel of intellect, image, and appearances that I had been schooled in.

First I went to Berkeley, where I stayed with a friend and tried to earn enough money to take a workshop at Esalen. I didn't have to wait long because someone ran into my bus. I collected $400 insurance and sent it to Esalen for a two-week workshop in Gestalt and Structural Integration. I used to tell people that I was a particularly slow learner so I came for two weeks but it took me five years to get it. Anyhow, I got hired as a cook at the end of my workshop and I did stay for that long.

During the first three months of my Esalen stint, I received ten sessions of Rolfing—often with two and three Rolfers working on me at the same time. This procedure changed me. Before being Rolfed I experienced my body as a troublesome, awkward, unpredictable, painful (especially in the low back), and unforgiving taskmaster. As I was Rolfed in that initial series, my body evolved first from taskmaster to teacher, providing me with essential information. Then it became a colleague who was available for exchange of information, and finally was transformed into a friend who was awfully fussy but dependable.

This process profoundly affected my mind, body, and spirit, but I will save that description for another day.

A couple of years after being Rolfed, and while still at Esalen, I decided that I, too, wanted to be a Rolfer. I had spent the previous nine months studying to be a psychotherapist with a psychologist (and recently trained Rolfer) named William C. Schutz. I soon realized that Will had a particular vision and dimension of understanding that I lacked and that he couldn't really teach me. I knew it had something to do with his Rolfer's view of the body. What he had, I wanted.

In the two years I had been at Esalen, I had studied/experienced a full spectrum of different techniques and therapies, including many body disciplines such as Reichian therapy, yoga, reflexology, and massage. Yet I remained frustrated because I still couldn't see the body the way these Rolfers did. I was certain that if I could become a Rolfer, it would give me the grounding in body physiology that I had been unable to acquire up to that point. I sent in an application to the newly formed Rolf Institute in Boulder, Colorado, submitted the required paper, and scheduled for an interview with Dr. Rolf and something called The Selection Committee. I felt calm and sanguine that Dr. Rolf would see me as an excellent candidate for her training . . . yet I had heard stories.

The day of my interview, I walked into a room in the Joe Adams House at Esalen, and there, situated in a tight semicircle, were six Rolfers (many of whom I knew) with this lovely if somewhat austere Victorian lady right in the center. I sat down and Ida Rolf began to speak.

"Well, Jason," she began, "your paper is acceptable and you do come to us with good references from the Esalen Rolfers. I understand from all of this that you would like to become a Rolfer." My memory is that before I could squeeze out a reply she went right on. "Let's see, it says here that you graduated from Harvard a few years ago and that in the intervening time you have studied and led Encounter and Gestalt Therapy groups, practiced t'ai chi ch'uan, and taken workshops in the Feldenkrais Method, Psychosynthesis, massage, Bioenergetics, yoga, meditation, and the Arica training, among others."

I sat back and tried to appear modest and demure while thinking, "Yeah, you really have accomplished a lot, after all. Hell, she's not as tough as people said. This is going to be easy." "Yes, Dr. Rolf," I said diffidently, "I have tried to make good use of the two and a half years that I have been here at Esalen." "Well, I think that is admirable, Jason, and I want to commend you for your efforts," she said. At some point I started to daydream a little about why the other

Rolfers were even there. This was clearly her show and I was in. I wondered how soon I could train—spring or summer would be OK. "Well, Jason," I thought I heard her say, "I really want to thank you for taking the time to apply, write your paper, and come in to see us. I really enjoyed meeting you but you'll never be a Rolfer."

I was sure I had misunderstood her, so I didn't say anything, not wanting to appear foolish. "Well, Jason," she continued, "we have several other people to interview today. So thank you again for coming in, and I do hope that I'll have a chance to visit with you again one day." Then it got through to me. She had rejected me. My God, she was blowing me off. "Excuse me, Dr. Rolf. I really do want to be a Rolfer. Is there something that I've done or something that you see that makes you think that I would not be a good candidate?" "Jason," she said, "we are interested in having practitioners who bring a level of focus and commitment to this work that is one-pointed and exclusive of other disciplines. We really don't have time or interest in training a Human Potential dilettante."

Well, my sweet ones, if she had stood up and thrown a mud pie in my face, I wouldn't have been any more shocked or stunned. "But, Dr. Rolf," I stammered, "I'm not a dilettante." (I wasn't really sure what a dilettante was but I knew it wasn't good.)

"I'm really serious about Rolfing." "Yes, yes," she went on, "of course you are. But I'm afraid that you will never be a Rolfer. Thank you very much. And on your way out, would you please send in the next person?"

"Well, the hell with her," I thought. "I've worked too hard. I want this too much. I'm not leaving until she says yes!" I stayed right there making my case, pleading really. "Dr. Rolf, I have all the qualifications that you require and I really want to be a Rolfer." At this she became irritated, saying, "Jason, how many times do I have to tell you? You will never, ever be a Rolfer. Please leave this room." But I wouldn't and I didn't. I could be just as obstinate as she was. What was it about this old lady? I really did want to be a Rolfer. Actually I wanted it more than I had ever wanted anything—more than getting into a good college, more than marrying my girlfriend, more than becoming another Will Schutz. . . . What was she doing to me?

So, there I stayed—mute and intractable. The other Rolfers in the room were fidgeting by this time and looked as uncomfortable as I felt. She broke the silence and said downright venomously, "Oh, Jason, come over here." Obediently, I stood up and walked over to her. "Let me see your hands." After studying, squeezing, and feeling my hands like she was trying to find a ripe piece of fruit, she said, "Your hands are OK. But Jason, you're just too much in your head. If you really want to pursue our training any further then I want you to complete a thousand-hour certification course in massage and go build something with those hands. Get out of that head of yours and maybe we can talk again. Now, good luck and good-bye!"

I decided to accept this pathetic and confusing crumb she had thrown at me and left the room. For the rest of the afternoon, children, I was in a fog, actually more like a stupor. I had never experienced anything or anyone quite like this before. I marched off to see Beverly Silverman, one of the Rolfers in attendance, and sniveled, "Beverly, what was that? Why won't she train me?" "Don't worry, Jason," Beverly said with unwarranted reassurance, "she liked you. Just do what she asked you to do, and see what happens." "Easy for her to say," I thought, "She was allowed to train with only a minimum of massage instruction and now I have to put in a thousand hours and 'build something,' whatever that means." Beverly told me that there was a thousand-hour massage school in Berkeley taught by Gunvar and Keith Jackson and that I could commute from Big Sur.

So that was that. I spent the next several months

driving from Big Sur to Berkeley and back in order to take this punitively long massage course. (Of course I learned a great deal from this course and did get much more in touch with my body.) The following summer, I went back East to Cape Cod and worked with my hands in a boatyard, sanding, painting, and doing light carpentry. By summer's end, I was proud that I could paint a straight, clean water line on any boat in the yard.

Subsequently, over a year after my original interview, I went to Los Angeles for another Selection Committee meeting. This time I knocked very softly on the door and tried to transform my terror into pure energy. A part of me was sure that all my efforts were completely in vain and that I had been a total idiot to do what she suggested.

"Come on in, Jason," I heard her say, "it's good to see you again. Now, let us have a look at you. Well, your body looks much better. You do look sturdier and your structure seems more stable and organized. I see from your file that you have completed the thousand-hour massage course and worked with your hands last summer in a boat yard. Now, we do have a class in Boulder next month that has space for another auditor, or there is a fall class in San Francisco. Which would best suit your needs and schedule?"

That was my first experience with Ida Rolf. Later I heard her say that Rolfers need to learn to walk on shifting sands. I had begun to learn this lesson. With this experience, she taught me that I could be tough and resolute with all my precious and newly acquired sensitivity, and that by being brought to my knees I could learn to persevere and hold my head up high.

Now we'll fast forward to June of 1979, when you will find me in the first week of an advanced Rolfing training in Philadelphia, Pennsylvania. You can imagine this is the first week of our working with "models," who are people who pay a reduced fee and come in to be a kind of guinea pig for a Rolfer in training. That first day of class, I was in the middle of performing a first session (of the ten-session series) on my model. During this initial session I was trying to develop rapport with my model, and you should remember that I had been a successful Rolfer with a full practice for the past five years and had a high level of confidence in my work.

Suddenly from somewhere behind me I heard this voice practically screaming, "Get that Rolfer off that poor model." I was certain she couldn't be talking to me so I just kept working. Dr. Rolf said, "Jason,

Jason, stop what you're doing." And I said, "Yes, Dr. Rolf." She said, "Who taught you to Rolf?" "Well, Emmett Hutchins and Peter Melchior, Dr. Rolf." "I don't believe it," she said. "You climb off of that poor model and let another Rolfer complete the session. I'm not going to have you take him apart."

So here it was again. This time I had more confidence than five years before, so I went into the kitchen and I thought to myself, "That miserable old lady! What right does she have to humiliate me in front of my classmates and in front of my model, after I have worked so hard practicing her method? I'm not going to take this. I don't need this. I'm leaving. There's no way I'm going to sit still for eight weeks of this."

Then Andy Crow, assistant to the class, came in and asked me how I was doing. He said, "Well, that must have been a little rough for you in there." "Andy," I said, "rough hardly describes it. She was insulting, humiliating, and I'm not going to take it. I'm out of here. I'm going home to my nice little practice in Carmel and say to hell with this. To hell with you. To hell with the advanced training and to hell with her!" I was, as they say in psychology, highly reactive.

Andy said emphatically, "Jason, I want you to do something for me. Stay the week, and if you want to

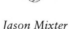

leave at the end of the week, leave. You'll have my complete support and I'll do everything I can to get you a refund. Just stay till the end of the week and see what happens. Actually, I think she likes you and this may be how she is showing her affection."

"Well, that may be, Andy, but I don't feel any affection. I just feel blah blah blah blah," and I went into a tirade. At any rate, Andy did talk me into staying. With a sullen and resentful countenance I went back into the classroom. Dr. Rolf didn't give me so much as a glance. I sat over on the side and watched my fellow student Rolfer work on my model. I felt like Tom Thumb, about two inches high.

After lunch, when we were all together without our models, Dr. Rolf was lecturing. She turned to the class and said, "I guess I was a little hard on Jason this morning." Inside I was going, "A little hard— you don't know what a little hard is. You were vicious, cruel, humiliating. . . ." Then she betrayed a little twinkle in her eye. She turned and looked completely away from me and said, "You know, the Lord chasteneth whom he loveth."

Well, that did it. I immediately soared from the deepest valley of despair to the highest peak of euphoria. I didn't leave the class and I did complete the advanced training. In fact, Dr. Rolf and I developed a close relationship, not as close as some, but close

Remembering Ida Rolf

enough for me. I came to realize how pathetically vulnerable I was to the ever-changing judgments of those to whom I gave power. I was like a feather floating along the capricious currents of other people's opinions. If the wind blew down, I went down with it. If the wind blew up, I went up. In fact, I had very little "center."

Since that day, I have worked hard to develop more of a center within myself, one which is increasingly able to withstand the vagaries of external opinions. This, by the way, is called self referral, while my former state was one of object (other people) referral. I sincerely hope that you, during the labyrinthian course of your journey here, learn way before I did to value your own judgments and opinions—not in exception to but in addition to those of others, no matter how powerful, wise, and respected they may appear to be.

The last thing I want to tell you about this remarkable woman occurred toward the end of the same advanced class. Dr. Rolf had been suffering from colon cancer for quite some time. None of us knew how serious her disease was and/or how much longer she had to live. Of course, we were all very concerned.

She had lost much of her eyesight, so a few of us used to go out to her apartment on weekends to read to her.

I remember the first day I walked into her modest Blackwood, New Jersey, apartment. She said "Now, Jason, there are six different kinds of chairs in this living room. I want you to sit in every one of them and find the one that fits your structure the best." Well, I was tall and had always had a vulnerable lower back, and so I did as she suggested and found a chair that was comfortable and with a seat at an appropriate height. In all of the living rooms that I had visited up to that point in time, no one had ever made an offer like this. And it really made a difference. I felt a lot better sitting in a chair that didn't cause my pelvis to tip back and squeeze my lower back.

Anyhow, I read to Dr. Rolf. I read Capra's *The Tao of Physics,* Agatha Christie mystery novels, articles from the *Scientific American,* and I think some of Carlos Castaneda's books about the teachings of Don Juan. She was a voracious learner, and loved taking in information of any kind.

One day while I was reading to her she said, "You know, Jason, I have colon cancer." "Yes, Dr. Rolf," I said awkwardly, "I understand that you do. I'm terribly sorry and I hope it's not giving you too much pain." "It's not too bad," she said, "but, you know, these New York Rolfers have a healer they want me to see. They think he can help me." "Dr. Rolf, maybe you should go see this person," I said quickly. "Maybe he or she can help." "No, no, no," she said, "I know healers that are much better than these boys."

So now I was hooked. I looked over at this silver-haired legacy whom I respected, occasionally hated, had learned so much from in all areas of life, and had finally come to love, telling me that she knew people that she believed could heal her. "Dr. Rolf, if you know healers that are better than the ones here, let's go to them. I'll take you there right now or any time you say." "No, no, no" (three of her most favorite words, by the way), "I've completed my assignment here. I just want to know what my next assignment is."

It has taken many years for me to appreciate fully the implications of this last comment, but even then I knew that I had just heard something important and personally transforming. Until that point, my Western reductionist, scientific mind really believed that we were all here as random events and that it was just a matter of luck who she was, who I was, and who anybody was. After all, my grandfather (and his father before him) was a well-known surgeon at the Massachusetts General Hospital, and I was named after him and born to continue the tradition. I, too, should have been a surgeon. Now, it was nice that I was a Rolfer, and I was glad to have found something that seemed to nourish myself as well as others, but fundamentally I was still a failure who had missed what I was supposed to have done in this life and would forever have to settle for mediocrity and second best.

But what was it she said? Something about an assignment? Now let's examine this. Is it my assignment to be right here, reading to her, a student of her work, not making anywhere near the kind of money I thought that I should make? Hmmm. Does that mean this whole thing is exactly the way it is supposed to be? Instead of being a mistake, what if I (and everyone) were here through some sort of divine appointment? OK. Now just supposing that's the case, what does that tell us about why we're here? What's our job? Well, maybe our job is simply to do our assignment. Not some movie star's assignment, or prominent relative's assignment, not some fantasy husband or fantasy wife's assignment, but our own individual assignment. What's the one thing that no one else can do except me? The one assigned to me. I'm telling you, kids, this understanding rocked my world and continues to change my life on many levels.

There is the teleological notion that I am here and you are here in order to serve a higher purpose. Although I had long believed this to be true, it was an intellectual belief that was in conflict with my heart and emotions. Sometime later I learned that the Vedic scriptures (from India) say each of us has his or her own Dharma, our own individual purpose for being here. This is something that we can do that no one else on the planet can do as well, as completely, as competently, or as successfully. According to this teaching, the goal of life is not to attain success according to someone else's prescription, not to earn the most money just for its own sake or to have the biggest reputation, the most friends, etc. The goal of life, on the contrary, is to discover your Dharma, your assignment, and to get busy working on it.

So, my sweet ones, if you can hear any of what I am saying, please hear this. You are here only to discover what your assignment, what your Dharma is. Listen to others with more experience than you for their counsel and advice, but don't let them tell you what you're supposed to do or how you're supposed to do it. That is for you to discover and for you alone. Take Dr. Rolf's perspective to heart and let it be a guide and comfort to you as it has been for me.

So there it is. There's so much more I could tell you about this remarkable woman, but I hope these few remembrances will spark something in you as they have in me. She was fundamentally a whole person without pretense and with few limitations. She could be on one hand inaccessible and elitist, unreasonable, demanding, and abrasive. And, yet, she was extraordinary—charming, witty, wise, intuitive, compassionate, and inspirational. And as she reached the end of her duties here she consciously lay down and transcended her physical vehicle, leaving us wiser, sturdier, more self-reliant, and with a fresh and enduring line of inquiry. She was born 100 years ago this year and I hope you will join me in wishing her a very Happy Birthday and good luck with the next assignment.

I love each of you very much, and remember Dr. Rolf's gift to Daddy and maybe to you, too: Don't let anybody tell you who you are or why you're here—even me.

Love,
Daddy

Dorothy Hunter

In 1974 I took a leave of absence from my IBM/Cape Kennedy job and traveled with my friend Michael to Santa Monica where Michael was to take his advanced training with Ida, to be preceded by auditing the beginning class. It was to be a long stay in California—three months! My thought was to go hang out with M. and perhaps get a job that would be really interesting . . . driving a truck or tending bar were what came to mind.

Anna Hyder approached me. Ida needed a secretary, a do-everything person. The pay was very low and the hours very long and I was a bit afraid of her. I had heard "stories." It was the "How could you possibly turn down a chance to be around Ida Rolf" that got me, so I agreed to take on the job.

Early on she found out that I had worked as a secretary and had somewhere in the far, far distant past taken shorthand. "Take a letter," she commanded. "But," my mind said, "it's been so long ago," as my fingers raced to do her bidding, pulling out of some dusty chamber of my mind those strange markings that could be transcribed into words. As I scribbled she would deliver these beautifully phrased letters without a pause, not one "strike that out" or "let me say that differently" or "change that." From beginning to end one seamless piece that always contained one charming phrase to set it off. I knew not one corporate executive who could have done it better.

Why this of all the memories I have of her sits on top, I do not know. Perhaps it's because those letters bring back to me her sharp intelligence, her organized mind, and her charm and sense of humor.

Allan Davidson, M.A.

When Ida was teaching in San Francisco in the early 1970s, she took a temporary apartment in a high-rise building. Soon after, Moshe Feldenkrais, also teaching in town, moved into the same building. When Ida was asked if she was aware that Moshe had moved in two floors below her, she replied, "Yes, and that's entirely appropriate."

At a question-and-answer session after a lecture-demonstration that Ida gave in Denver to a group of doctors and other medical professionals, a doctor from England asked (somewhat as follows), "Dr. Rolf, could you give us some perspective on the background of your work—how you came to put it together and who influenced you?" Ida fixed him with an icy stare and, after a long pause, said with a steely voice, "No." I don't think there were too many more questions after that.

Francis Wenger, M.D.
Anecdote of Dr. Rolf

Back in 1975, I learned about a technique called Rolfing or structural integration and an associated discipline called patterning from a brilliant sophomore medical student, Tom Findley, M.D., PH.D., now director of research at the Kessler Institute and at one time Chairman of Research for the Rolf Institute. I employed Rick Wheeler, now a Rolfer, to come to the Washington Hospital Center for a two-week course in patterning with my staff and one or two patients. We videotaped the whole thing and Judith Aston came at the end. Then I got Rolfed by the first practitioner in Washington and knew I had to understand this thing.

Dr. Rolf agreed to come for a lecture-demonstration at the hospital and I asked her if I could study Rolfing. "It will change your life," she said, but she must have agreed because I audited and trained in fast sequence. Dr. Rolf: "If you do it my way, you will get my results." Period. Being vastly afflicted with lower consciousness as an allopathic physician, I found that the careful nurturing and supervision of Sharon Wheeler-Hancoff opened new visions and kaleidoscopic involvement as part of the cadre of Rolfers about Dr. Rolf, from liaison with Buckminster Fuller to study with Moshe Feldenkrais. The Valerie Hunt study was just completed, and after meeting this group in California I presented a synopsis at the annual meeting of the Gardner Murphy Foundation for parapsychology.

Dr. Rolf grumpily said "Psychic phenomena is unexplained physics." However, she confided that in the 1920s she was in love with Gardner Murphy and he with her best girl friend. She gave me some confidential messages for him and the assignment of carrying them to him. At this time, Gardner Murphy was bedridden with Parkinson's disease and required daily nursing care. The only approach was through an undersecretary of HEW, a friend. I was finally invited to tea by his charming wife. There was a blizzard that day; I abandoned my car and hiked through the snow up a hill. The nurse could not make it, so I nursed him that day and delivered my messages. At more than ninety he was still one of the most structurally perfect humans I have ever seen. Gardner Murphy died on March 3rd and Dr. Rolf on March 4th, 1979.

Nicholas French

I've heard people describe Ida as frightening and/or infuriating. Perhaps she was mellowing by the time I studied with her, for I found her to be brilliant, tough and demanding, but also loving (in a non-huggy, Zen master sort of way), compassionate, and very funny. She could be tender as well as exacting, and was extraordinarily respectful of people.

In one class, she selected me as a person who needed work around the ischial rami. The manner of the work at one point was for me to stand, with an advanced class student kneeling on each side of me, each with a hand reaching up into the tissue around each ramus. They were to lift; I was to lengthen along the inner line so as to keep my feet on the ground. I groaned and sweated, but would not allow myself to curse as I ordinarily would. After all, the Victorian lady was watching closely. It was a painful but very powerful session. After the break, I sat down, spacy as I was, to hear her lecture. Ida insisted I lie down and rest. I lay on a mat, another student covered me, and I was out in a second. Later, I was told that during her lecture she heard me snoring, and said, "He worked hard—he deserves the rest."

One day I was asked to take by Ida's house a couple of loaves of bread she was fond of. At the door, her companion told Ida that I was at the door. Ida wanted me to come in and talk with her. While she ate lunch (and groused about the food), we chatted about class, Rolfing, the relative merits of endomorphs and mesomorphs. Suddenly, she asked what was on my mind. "Well, you're getting pretty old," I said. "Yes, I am," she replied.

"You aren't going to live much longer," I muttered. "No, not much longer," she said. "You know, there are a lot of people who'd probably be willing to take a year off their lives to give to you," I ventured. She smiled, "I know, but I don't want them. I'm tired, and I want a rest."

When I finally left, I wished her whatever she wanted for however long she wanted. She said, "Thank you, kind sir," and though seated, did a sort of formal curtsy.

Another day toward the end of my practitioning class, I went to her morning lecture feeling weird and spacy. Therefore, I sat well over to the side of the class, where I was relatively sure she couldn't see me and call on me to answer a question. Halfway into the lecture, I began to experience a phenomenon I'd known as a child and which had frightened me. I was hearing what Ida was about to say, as well as what she was saying. The effect was very disorienting, like hearing the same soundtrack, but one with a delay of a couple of seconds. As a child, I'd stopped it—and here it was again. I was sure I was cracking up.

Suddenly Ida stopped in mid-sentence, turned and looked straight at me, and asked, "What's on your mind?" I had the clear sense I'd just been caught eavesdropping. I had no idea what to say—"Uh . . . well, uh. . . ."

She grinned and waved her hand at me. "Don't worry, it's just a quantum leap in your spiritual process. Nothing to be afraid of, you'll be fine." And she turned back and picked up her lecture in mid-sentence, and went right on.

Now I was certain I was losing it—an hallucination, obviously. But at the break, some of the other students came up and asked me what the hell happened. When I asked what they meant (not wanting to show my craziness any more than necessary) they went through the event word for word, just as I'd heard it myself.

At the end of the class, sitting alone with Ida, there she was looking at me again while I felt uncertain how to say what I felt. Finally I told her I wanted to thank her for what she'd given us—and I just didn't know how to express my gratitude adequately. She smiled and said softly, "Go out there and get to work."

The final day of class, partly on a dare, when I went to say goodbye to Ida, I shook her right hand, but also took hold of her left hand—to prevent her from possibly hitting me—as I bent over and kissed her on the cheek. It was as soft as any cheek I've ever touched. She said something like "Oh, go on with you . . ." And she blushed right down to her roots.

Ida would sometimes come down the hill to class late, and one of her assistants would have gotten us started on discussing some aspect of the work. It was observed, fairly often, that when she arrived and made herself comfortable, she would pick up on the subject where we'd stopped and build her lecture on that point. And no one had told her what we'd been talking about. Curious. . . .

On the first day of our combined basic and advanced class, Ida asked us to define "energy." Most of us tried. Some of us sounded pretty brilliant, I thought. But Ida just shook her head and told us we obviously didn't know what we were talking about. She chose to address her remarks to the last student who'd spoken, and seemed to be really chewing him out, telling him he needed to look further, that "the roadmap is not the territory." He took the rebuke well, while the rest of us cringed, glad we weren't him.

On the last day of that class, she asked that student to stand. She reminded us of the first day's exchange, and then thanked him for letting her use him to make the point to the rest of us. It was suddenly obvious that she'd chosen someone who was dialectically strong to use as a lightning rod. She somehow knew he wouldn't feel injured by her words.

Tom Myers

Ida Rolf first entered my life in Boulder in 1978, when friends from my Arica training would return with literal red welts on their bodies, yet raving about their "Rolfing" sessions. A fellow Arican (it was then a full-immersion spiritual training cult, now very different) who later became a fellow itinerant Rolfer tried to show me what they were experiencing by putting his fists on my chest and seemingly flaying the skin off my ribs. My teeth tingled and my breathing was immediately easier. "Far out!"

So when I heard, in early '74, that Ida Rolf was giving a class and needed mod ls for students to work on (for cheap), I hurried to sign up. By this time I had an enviably silly job in the rock 'n roll paradise that was the Hollywood hills in the mid-1970s, and thought I was pretty hot shit. I showed up at the appropriate hour, but while I was filling out the MMPI that some UC students were using to study Rolfing's personality effects, I was told that I was the one-too-many model, and could not participate in the class. A brief tantrum raised the eyebrows of Ida's secretary, Jane Hale, who was back in a few minutes saying that Jan Sultan, Ida's assistant, would Rolf me (for not quite so cheap) after hours.

Shortly after Ida Rolf came in and began her talk. You have pictures of her, so you have no need of my description—the terrible posture, the unbreakable face. What doesn't come across in a photo is the academic diction with a Jersey accent. Some author was there that day, of some wildly popular and long-forgotten self-help book, and as usual she played to him, and as usual when she was defending against some yet-to-appear attack on her work, she brayed. I have no memory of what she said that day, only the face, voice, eyes, and hands, and the feeling of having met someone who had accomplished something real at some undefined cost to herself.

My housemate Steve had come with me to this talk and Ida chose him as her model. Steve was one of those strong but consumptive types whose front was so close to his back that from the side he could barely be seen. In one hour of what she called "processing," Ida Rolf gave his chest depth, depth which I can attest lasted for some months even though Steve always put off going for more sessions. As he stood up, his ribs moving with his breath, I recall thinking, "This is useful magic."

After the demo, I went to ask Dr. Rolf a question in my usual "first in the class" manner. The night before I had gone to see another luminary of the then-current human potential scene, a fellow with the unlikely name of Werner Erhard who was perhaps the funniest stand-up comic I had ever seen. One of his many points was that while recipients of Nobel Prizes often had gray hair, the moment of creative inspiration that drove the work that got them the prize usually came in their twenties, and the ensuing years were the perspiration that finally resulted in recognition. Now here, the very next day, I had run across, well, not a Nobel Prize winner, but certainly an innovator. So I asked her something like, "Did you have your original inspiration for this work in your twenties, and everything after has been more or less an elaboration?"

I knew later that personal questions and especially anything that suggested she was not as creative at seventy-eight as she was at twenty-eight were most unwelcome. I crawled away from her indignant sputter feeling about two inches tall, and swearing that I would never ask that old lady another question, a promise I was not to keep.

So I was Rolfed after hours by Jan in front of several students, who stayed after to watch him work, and most interestingly for me, to ask the questions they dared not ask when Ida was around. Between Jan's fingers of steel and my uptight Puritan background, I spent most of these sessions in hyperventilation tetany, but I was fascinated by both the physical and psychic effects of the sessions, and the students' questions gave me some idea of the intellectual system out of which they grew.

Toward the end of my sessions, I asked Jan about becoming a Rolfer. Tired probably, of trying to get my tautly strung puerile body into another shape, he replied, "Don't even try, you won't make it in." It took me two years to prove him wrong. Within weeks I quit the cushy job and headed off to the Bay Area for massage school and anatomy and physiology courses, the start of my career as a Rolfer.

I saw Ida Rolf only once more before I began training with her—at a Rolfers' conference in Mill Valley. During a question-and-answer period, I stood up and asked, "When I am trained as a Rolfer, where should I go?" "Young man," she intoned, "you can go anywhere. Go where there are no Rolfers and spread the gospel." Prophetic words; during the late 1970s and 1980s, I was to open practices in eight cities in the United States and Europe where there were no practitioners, and was always able to pass on the practice to one or two others as I left.

Observation at some distance had given me a

better understanding of her nature. Before I came to train with her I found, framed, and sent her an illuminated quote from Thomas Browne—"Those who undertake great public schemes must be prepared for the most fatiguing delays, mortifying disappointments, and worst of all, the presumptuous judgment of the ignorant upon his design." When she met me after that, she gave me the once-over and said, "So you're Tom Myers, I expected someone older." Sometime later I came across Ecclesiastes 7:29: "Lo, this only have I found that the Lord hath made man upright and straightforward, but he hath sought out many directions of his own." I had this printed up also and sent to her, but it was received without comment.

I attended her gala eightieth birthday at the San Francisco Yacht Club, but my only memory of the evening is Moshe Feldenkrais showing up (in the same clothes he had been wearing all day, perhaps all year), and Dr. Rolf, in her finery. She was both pleased and uncomfortable with all this attention and gratefully seized him. They spent the next hour or more huddled over a small table, backs to the rest of the celebrants, talking about God knows what.

Like the old farmer in the Taoist story, I never know what's lucky and what's unlucky. Delays plagued my impatient path to become a Rolf practitioner, but the happy result was that finally in 1976 I got to practition with Ida Rolf. I was a neophyte, and we were folded into an advanced class she was giving. She would hold forth and give a demonstration in the morning, and we would go off on our own for the afternoon to be taught the basics by Peter Melchior, her laconic, Indian-like second-in-command.

Anatomy from the diffident Louis Schultz, PH.D., movement from the definite Judith Aston—I was too young yet to know how short these days would be, how lucky I was to be so near source. Ida was by now in her early eighties and would sometimes assign the work of the demonstration to Peter, though her watchful eye never left his hands, and her crooked admonitory finger hovered constantly.

One rather sickly child came in for a session. After working on her, Ida took the parents off into a corner where I happened to have my nose in a book and recommended, "That child needs some Phlogiston 4." The parents nodded earnestly, but I doubt they were able to find it; the phlogiston theory has been well out of favor for fifty years.

Another time one of my fellow practitioners, Nicholas French, had a session in class. After the session, he was sitting and listening to the lecture, when Ida said rather suddenly and sharply to him, "Don't you need to sleep?" Within minutes, Nicholas was snoring away in the back of the classroom, and Dr. Rolf simply raised her voice a few decibels without complaint.

Her main model for this class was a boy named Logan. These sessions were videotaped and survive in the Institute archives. Logan was twelve and a heavy walker. Dr. Rolf did a "lower eighth"—a pelvic girdle session—which would dictate an "upper ninth"—a shoulder girdle session—according to her own system. She spent the next morning railing against us, abjuring us in the harshest stentorian tones that "If we do a lower eighth we must do an upper ninth"— and vice versa—while Logan stood uncomfortably in his underwear on top of the Rolfing table. Then he lay down and she got down to work—a lower ninth, another session around his pelvis and legs. The lesson is lost on those who only watch the tapes.

During the class, another Rolfer called in from Little Rock, Arkansas—he had been traveling there and was now ready to stop; he had a full practice going begging; would anybody in the class want to take it? Dr. Rolf had a soft spot in her heart for Little Rock: an architect and student of hers had brought her there in the old days to work on people, and she remembered standing on the grassy runway outside of town to literally flag down the plane going from Memphis to Houston.

I wanted points with Ida Rolf; I had been thinking of going to Boston, but I said I would take the job. "Give this young man extra training, there are no Rolfers within 500 miles of Little Rock, so he'll be out on his own," she said to the assistants, who sighed and grumbled, and would have ignored the suggestion had I not pestered them. The result was that I did half again as many model sessions as the others and had to soak my hands in hot water and Epsom salts each night to be able to return to the field of battle the next day.

This is not an Ida Rolf story, but in case it's of interest: When I arrived in Little Rock, $500 and an old Volvo to my name, I found to my horror that a "full practice" was three of his leftovers and two maybe sign-ups. But after an evening introduction and the departure of my predecessor, the phone started ringing: "I couldn't work with that sociopath Bob T., but you, you're a sweet fellow and I'd like to start my Rolfing." Little Rock was very good to me, a full practice and more for two years running, but then travel called to me. I made a similar phone call to the Institute, pleased that I could pass on a full practice. To my horror, my long waiting list dwindled to two or three before my successor Brent E. showed up. He was likewise penurious and stunned. I did what I could, but my air tickets were set. After I left, his

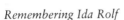

phone began to ring, "I never could stand that arro-
gant sonuvabitch Tom Myers, but you, you're soft
and accessible, I'd like to begin my Rolfing. . . ."

During my time in Little Rock, Ida Rolf's new
secretary Adrienne (she went through them like
Kleenex) called me up to get me to participate in an
advanced class. I demurred—I hadn't been working
long enough—you were supposed to have practiced
for at least three years; I had only been out there a
year and a half. She got Ida on the phone, who grudg-
ingly admitted that it would be all right if I came into
the class. It was only later that I learned that they
were desperate to fill that class and there were few
takers.

More luck for me, for it turned out to be Ida's last
class. By now eighty-three and being overtaken by
cancer, her body was failing fast and seriously. Her
mind was however still this sharp: Every morning we
would assemble in the back room of one of those thin
Philadelphia townhouses, and Andy Crow would
begin the class at nine, taking questions and promot-
ing discussion until Dr. Rolf showed up, sometime
before 9:30. Her arrival was announced by the clang-
ing of her wheelchair, the slamming of doors, and her
voice as she was settled into the wheelchair just so.
(Even at this late stage, her hair was always up and
always had a carnation in it. I saw her hair down

only once when I visited her early one day and
Adrienne was brushing it. It was long, white, and
smooth—what an Indian she looked that morning!)

"Energy," she would say, "You people don't understand en-er-gy" and she would start with William
Blake, go through Melville, cut back through
Maxwell and Van der Graaf, and take a bead on Ein-
stein, Planck, and Wiener. Aside from Bucky Fuller, I
have never met an intellect as wide.

Or as tough. This was, in fact, the first time I had
done more than a session or two in her presence, and
this non-perspirer had rings of underarm sweat under
her baleful eye. As a teacher, she was neither kind,
nor, in my experience, particularly helpful. I had had
a battle-ax of a grade school teacher in my two-room
elementary school, so this did not bother me much,
and she loved a good argument if you were up to it.

She tested whether you were up to it by ignoring
your first attempt at a question, belittling your second attempt, but often the third time around you felt
the searchlight of her intelligence creaking around to
bear on your question. Like Bucky, her sally into the
answer often seemed to come from so far out in left
field that you were sure she had misunderstood, until
she began to weave enough threads that the tapestry
began to reveal itself to you. I remember one such example: I was sitting in rapt attention on a treatment

table in front of her wheelchair while the others were in the kitchen on a break. She finished the pronouncements on the "objective" nature of Egyptian and Sumerian sculpture, and then before I could reply or even thank her: "Don't you feel how you are sitting on one sitz bone? If you keep that up, don't come crying to me about your sacrum." Discussion over.

One day someone was talking disparagingly about dowsing with a pendulum, and Dr. Rolf surprisingly jumped to its defense. Someone produced a chain with a bit of turquoise on the end, and I lay down on a treatment table. She held a chain over my various organs, coming up with the not surprising diagnosis (this was the late 1970s) that my "liver was out." Another student went to the hall and got his camera, and as he came back in to the room and lifted it to his eye, she saw him and snapped the pendulum up into her hand and handed it back. No one was going to have a record of the creator of Rolfing dowsing a patient.

For someone so scientific, she retained a keen interest in the psychic. During the advanced class, she would often call over the resident astrologer among the students and whisper in her ear, and the next morning Sydney would slip a worked-up chart to Ida.

She was not fond of the competition. It was a respectful rivalry with Feldenkrais, though his story of

Tom Myers

how they met at Bennett's place in the Cotswolds, which I got out of him as he dusted my car with cigarette ashes a few years later in London, was quite different from her version.

During that last Advanced class, I remember one break where a visitor asked her during a discussion of yoga and other body-changing techniques, "What about Alexander?" She looked the other way for a moment, then retorted, "I think he did a great job of conquering Egypt." End of discussion.

It was a friendly rivalry with Feldenkrais. Her version of their meeting in John Bennett's place in the Cotswolds, as it was told to me, had her giving a demonstration and inviting Feldenkrais up to the front so that he could make comments on what she was doing as she worked. According to her, he was so impressed that he undertook sessions with her.

But I got to hear his version as well, and this is how it came about: After Dr. Rolf died, I moved to London. One night I was invited to dinner in Hampstead by a client, a concert pianist. As so often with dinners in London, he had invited a specific group of people in order to set us hounds after a particular intellectual hare. The question for that night was, "Does one learn more through pleasure or through pain?" He had invited two psychiatrists from the Tavistock clinic, a Feldenkrais practitioner who was

220

visiting London, and myself. He expected (having had several of my sessions already) that the psychiatrists and the Feldenkrais practitioner would side with pleasure and I would side with pain. To all of our surprise, the psychiatrists voted for pain, with the Feldenkrais practitioner and myself taking the side of learning more from pleasure.

In the subsequent conversation, the Feldenkrais practitioner and I made fast friends. The next evening, she took me to meet Moshe. We decided to go to a movie, *Mon Oncle d'Amerique,* as I recall. On the way, cigarette ashes flying constantly around the car, he told me his version.

The beginning is the same—he commented on her demonstration—but in his version he was appalled that she could ask him for money. "Me! She called me one of her teachers!" Then he said something more interesting: "I came into her class on the last day and said, 'You know, my system is more powerful than your system.' 'Oh yes?' she said, 'Why is that?' 'Because my system allows me to learn from you, but your system doesn't allow you to learn from me.'" At that point, according to Moshe, Ida Rolf broke down and cried, saying that she didn't dare work with him in case it did replace her work. He remembers that she said, "I just can't give up what I have worked on so hard." Moshe went on to lament,

Tom Myers

"I made that strong woman cry—that was a bad thing. Nowadays I wouldn't do that."

I must say that the words he put in Ida's mouth do not sound like hers, but then Moshe was remembering an event about twenty-five years previous.

Though wearing glasses and a veteran of at least one cataract operation, Ida Rolf still possessed her unique way of seeing, even at this late date. I was bent over a treatment table with my hands underneath my supine client, searching his back muscles for an offending restriction. Dr. Rolf was behind me in her wheelchair, so she could see my back, and the client's head and feet. "Jack, Jack, it's under your ring finger." While I silently seethed that even after four years, she did not know my name, I probed in with my right ring finger. "No, no, the ring finger of your left hand." My irritation gave way to wonder as my left hand found the spindle-shaped fascicle that was holding his back in a curve.

Her hands may have lost strength, but not authority. A client from Little Rock had taken the trouble to travel to Philadelphia to be my model, and to have Ida Rolf's eyes on her extraordinarily scoliotic spine. A bustling nurse despite severe torquing of her spine and rib cage that had laid her spinous processes onto the transverse in several vertebrae, Tweed loved Rolfing for the energy it gave her, though curing the

Remembering Ida Rolf

curvature was beyond the scope of any manipulation.
I had her on a bench, and was going down her back
with my hands on either side as she rolled forward.
Ida Rolf was behind me, wanting me to (how often
she said this) "go deeper." There was something I was
not getting and finally her admonitory fingers got so
itchy that she locked the brake on the wheelchair,
reached out at full stretch, and brought two fingers
down Tweed's erectors. Tweed was still leaning forward, and unaware that I had stepped aside, said,
"That's it, now you're getting it." It was a revelatory
moment: After hearing it 490 times, the 491st I realized that going deeper was not the same as going
harder. That old woman can get deeper than I while
leaning way out of a wheelchair. . . .

It was during this class that I had my only work
at the hands of the founder of Rolfing. Although the
reputation for pain in Rolfing has been confirmed
many times, my own experience was that her touch
was gentle but commanding. The tissue of my mouth
and neck seemed to say, "You know, I was just going
this way anyway."

Early the next year Ida Rolf succumbed. I went to
visit her in a nursing home in Bryn Mawr, where she
waited out her last days. She had had a pacemaker
implanted, a step so out of tune with her character
that I wondered until I visited her and saw so clearly

what had been an unspoken perception before: There were two people in there, Ida and Dr. Rolf. Ida was mortally tired of this mortal coil, but Dr. Rolf would not let go until she knew that her legacy was safely in the hands of others; it was only a few days, as I understand it, from the conclusion of an agreement transferring the rights to Rolfing to the Rolf Institute until she let go into her death.

It was four days before she died that I stepped into her sunny, simple room. We talked a bit about this and that—I was about to leave for a trip to Europe, which was later to become my home. We talked about Switzerland and England, where she had studied and worked.

She was always interested in my family business of aquaculture. She said, "When you meet my husband, he'll tell you he has a great recipe for mussels, but don't you believe him, because he doesn't know what he's talking about." This and a few other statements showed that she was unstuck in time—her husband, an enigmatic figure at best, had been out of the picture for decades.

She was in and out, and I soon felt that she was using energy she sorely needed trying to be a good host to me. Her body was tiny, birdlike—only her large head and strong hands still held energy. I took one hand in mine, and gently kissed her forehead.

The other hand waved me away in weak protest, but she smiled. She passed into sleep, and four days later she was dead.

I have been in practice twenty years this year, and she is still very alive for me, though I have moved into many other explorations in the meantime. There is a Karsch photo of her used in every publication. It shows her in what I call her "grandmother" image—gentle, benign, ready for another sugar cookie with her second cup of tea. I find this part easy to remember, and not very inspiring.

Thus I was grateful to find, leafing through Curtis prints in a gallery in Santa Fe, the face of an old brave staring out through the century, one eye hooded, merciless, reptilian, the other looking through you toward a vision of a new way to live. Those were Ida's eyes, and below was her very face—hooked nose, the stubborn, determined set of her lips, even the hand visible in the corner was hers. This photo will not smile if I try to mix in trivial systems or lull myself with platitudes. It still occasionally provokes sweat, figuring out how she might approach what I am facing. We could use a few more like her, but I'm afraid they broke the mold.

Veronique Raskin
Requiem for a "Grande Dame"

New York City, October 1972, the wide stage of Carnegie Hall. A packed house here to see a white-haired lady, affectionately known as "the elbow," give a lecture. Rather stout and small, imperious in her gait and demeanor, she struts up and down the aisles, gesturing broadly in annoyance at the poor organization of the event. She is oblivious to the crowd, most of them young people, who watch her with a mixture of fearful reverence, friendliness, and surprise. The lecture starts, she is in great shape today. The formidable, inimitable grandma of the Human Potential Movement, none other than "Ida"—Dr. Ida P. Rolf.

This indomitable seventy-five-year-old doesn't just talk, she asserts authoritatively. It is clear that one does not argue with Ida, whose presence is unique. The audience is spellbound. They straighten their slouchy "in" postures for a while, impressed, convinced by what she is saying. She is a "Grande Dame."

Veronique Raskin

Tonight the audience looks at her with an expression I will almost always encounter on the faces of those who meet her. Instant affection, puzzlement, a being touched to the heart, a tenderness, desire to protect and care for her; and another feeling—awe, respect, sometimes fear. Ida does not leave anyone indifferent, that much is for sure.

The lecture is over. People crowd the stage and I, like others, feel compelled to seek contact with her. "Hello, Dr. Rolf," I say, bracing myself, for I have heard that she is quite abrasive, brutal sometimes in her answers, and that she brushes people off easily. I am uncomfortable, even though I stand a good head taller than she. "I am very interested in your method," I manage to mumble. "I wonder if you would let me attend one of your classes; I intend to write a PH.D. thesis on Rolfing and I need information." She sizes me up with her blue piercing eyes. "Show me your hands," she orders abruptly. Startled, I obey. How is that the answer to my question? She looks at my hands for an instant, then bluntly declares, "Your hands are too ladylike. You need peasant-type hands for this work. But your shoulders are okay. Write to us." She turns around and walks off. I stand there openmouthed, thunderstruck. Who on earth said I wanted to become a Rolfer? I don't qualify. It's man's work anyway.

But I am hooked, and I have the uncanny impression that I was "picked." I do not know yet just how much her search is my search, her work my work, viscerally so, almost as if she had invented it especially for me. And I am left with a strange déjà-vu feeling.

San Francisco, July 1977, the Yacht Club. A huge white room, candlelit and brimming with flowers, ours for this evening. The "family," the Rolf gang, is here for the annual meeting and to pay tribute to the old lady on her eightieth birthday. The "stars" of the "movement," Moshe Feldenkrais, her old buddy, and Werner Erhard, etc., circulate among the crowd of 300 celebrants.

Wheeled in, Ida Rolf is minute in her chair. She is dressed in white, looking as fragile as the red flower pinned in her white hair. The room lights are dimmed and all of us rise in unison and begin to sing "Happy Birthday" while a huge, radiant, candle-laden cake is brought in. My husband-to-be is here with me, astounded; he has never seen one single human being so loved, cherished, honored. This was Ida.

The spirit that now fills the room is not the adoration reserved for a religious leader, but rather a very unique kind of affection. Men and women, old-timers, beginners, all feel it. Ida possesses the uncanny ability to awaken this particular feeling in those who crossed her path. One may hold opposing views, argue with her teaching, note her faults (quite a few of them), but one's general response remains one of respect and tenderness. This is in part due to her age and appearance, as well as her personality and charm. But the truth is that we love this woman because her work has transformed our lives. For this reason a family feeling unites us.

Tonight we know that she is not well and getting weaker. All 300 of us beam out to her tenderness and healing energy. But Ida, typically, cuts it short. We know that she loves it but is most embarrassed by this kind of demonstration. So, over the years we have learned to express our affection on the sly, bringing her a cup of tea or a cookie in class, for instance, or a flower, a picture, small presents that she deigns to accept. Tonight, once more, she uses humor to cut us short. But we laugh and are not taken aback.

San Francisco, March 1979. Ida's condition has progressively worsened over the past few months. She has long been diabetic, then developed cancer of the intestine. The last time I saw her, she appeared tired of fighting. The time for her "final rest" was fast approaching, she said. But what about us? What would become of us without her? She who had founded our school, our family. To our fear is added the grief of losing a beloved. We pray therefore and avidly search for therapies likely to keep her with us a little while longer.

But she? She has had it. And if we really loved her, she points out, we would respect her desire to die. But the heart is hard pressed to practice such wisdom.

One day, for some obscure reason, I feel like calling her up. She's in a hospital on the East Coast recuperating from surgery. I finally reach her secretary, who explains that Dr. Rolf is too weak to speak. She assures me that she will transmit my "get well" wishes. I accept her decision and ring off. Then, impulsiveness overcoming reason, I call again. Would she do me a big favor? Would she please put the receiver next to Ida's ear? The secretary hesitates. I do realize, don't I, that Ida cannot respond. She may not even be able to hear me? Yes, I know, and that's all right with me. This is for me, so that I have the satisfaction of expressing my affection, my feelings. The secretary relents. The receiver goes silent. Profoundly moved, I manage to mumble, "Dr. Rolf, this is

Veronique. I just wanted to tell you . . . to remind you . . . just how . . . grateful we are to you . . . and . . . we love you."

Words strangle in my throat. I have never had the guts to tell her this straight to her face. Even now I note that I used "we" when it is *my* heart brimming over with tenderness. Surprised, the secretary intervenes again. Dr. Rolf has indicated that she got the message. I breathe a sigh of relief and joy, and I go back to work. We all know that it is only a matter of time, a few months at the most.

A quarter of an hour later, the telephone rings. The executive director of the Rolf Institute is on the line from Colorado. "Guess what," I say, "I just talked to Ida. And I even managed to slip an 'I love you' in the old lady's ear. Now what do you say to that?" Dick already knows; he calls to tell me that Ida died within a few minutes after my phone call.

Incredulous, I sit down and cry. But tempering my grief is the knowledge that she departed on a message of love. I am proud to have conquered my fear of "bothering her." Although stunned and grieving, in a strange way I am happy, and marveling at the synchronicity of events.

Reprinted with permission from *Guild Online,* 1992.